Manual on
Shirish Sheth
Vaginal Surgery

AF520942

68th All India Congress of Obstetrics & Gynaecology

aicog Delhi 2026

Advocate Innovate Challenge Optimise Globalise

Manual on *Shirish Sheth* Vaginal Surgery

Series Editors

Ashok Kumar
MD PhD
Director–Professor
Department of Obstetrics and Gynecology
Atal Bihari Vajpayee Institute of Medical Sciences
and Dr Ram Manohar Lohia Hospital
New Delhi, India

Madhavi M Gupta
MS
Director–Professor
Department of Obstetrics and Gynecology
Maulana Azad Medical College and Lok Nayak Hospital
New Delhi, India

K Aparna Sharma
MBBS MD
Professor
Department of Obstetrics and Gynecology
All India Institute of Medical Sciences
New Delhi, India

Editors

Rajendra Saraogi
Suman Sinha
Meenakshi
Nishi Makhija

JAYPEE

JAYPEE BROTHERS MEDICAL PUBLISHERS
The Health Sciences Publisher
New Delhi | London

Message from Series Editors

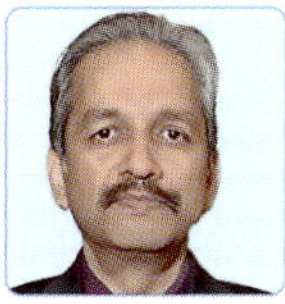

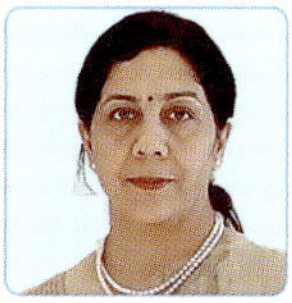

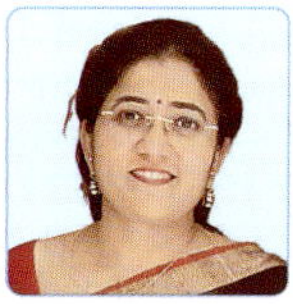

Ashok Kumar
Organizing Chairperson
AICOG-2026
New Delhi

Madhavi M Gupta
Organizing Secretary
AICOG-2026
New Delhi

K Aparna Sharma
Organizing Secretary
AICOG-2026
New Delhi

It is after 18 long years that the 68th AICOG is being held in New Delhi. It is a pleasure to welcome you all.

The Organizing Team have poured their heart and soul into curating an academic program which one will feel a loss if missed. The scientific sessions include both national and international faculty who are stalwarts in their fields. There are 18 workshops with 8 full-day and 5 each in the pre-lunch and post-lunch time.

On this occasion, the workshop faculty, have gone that extra mile to publish the workshop manual for eight workshops. This includes all recent scientific evidence and clinical management guidelines. These manuals will serve as a go-to evidence-based resource in your day-to-day clinical practice. We look forward to receiving your valuable feedback.

We acknowledge the hard work put in by all the editors, co-editors, and the authors, who, in spite of busy schedules and time constraints, have contributed immensely.

We would also like to thank M/s Jaypee Brothers Medical Publishers (P) Ltd, New Delhi, India, for partnering with us.

We sincerely hope that you will enjoy reading these manuals, find this manual useful, and treasure it for future use in your practical work.

We take this opportunity to wish you a memorable time during your stay in New Delhi.

Warm Regards

Jaypee Brothers Medical Publishers (P) Ltd

Headquarters
EMCA House, 23/23-B
Ansari Road, Daryaganj
New Delhi 110 002, India
Landline: +91-11-23272143, +91-11-23272703
+91-11-23282021, +91-11-23245672
e-mail: jaypee@jaypeebrothers.com

Corporate Office
4838/24, Ansari Road, Daryaganj
New Delhi 110 002, India
Phone: +91-11-43574357
Fax: +91-11-43574314
e-mail: jaypee@jaypeebrothers.com

Overseas Office
JP Medical Ltd.
83, Victoria Street, London
SW1H 0HW (UK)
Phone: +44-20 3170 8910
e-mail: info@jpmedpub.com

EU GPSR Authorised Representative
Logos Europe, 9 rue Nicolas Poussin
17000, La Rochelle, France
Phone: +33 (0) 6 67 93 73 78
e-mail: contact@logoseurope.eu

Website: www.jaypeebrothers.com
Website: www.jaypeedigital.com

Inquiries for bulk sales may be solicited at: jaypee@jaypeebrothers.com

Manual on Shirish Sheth: Vaginal Surgery

First Edition: **2026**

ISBN: 978-93-7545-883-8

Printed at: Samrat Offset Pvt. Ltd.

Contributors

Aarti Chitkara MBBS MD DNB
Consultant
Department of Obstetrics
and Gynecology
Eros Hospital
Karnal, Haryana, India

Ajay Aggarwal MBBS MD DNB
Director
Department of Obstetrics
and Gynecology
Amayra Healthcare
Chandigarh, India

Anil Sakhare MBBS DGO DFP DNB FICOG
Consultant
Department of Obstetrics
and Gynecology
Rayat Hospital
Nanded, Maharashtra, India

Ashok Kumar Todani MBBS DGO
Director
Department of Sonography Clinic
and Laparoscopy Centre
Bardhaman, West Bengal, India

Elizabeth Jacob MBBS DGO DNB
Head and Senior Consultant
Department of Obstetrics
and Gynecology
Apollo Adlux Hospital
Angamaly, Kerala, India

Ganpat Sawant
MD DGO FCPS DFP DNB DICOG
Former Head and Professor
Department of Obstetrics
and Gynecology
DY Patil Medical College, Navi Mumbai
Director
Noble and Noble Plus Hospital
Mumbai, Maharashtra, India

Juhi Agarwal MBBS MD FICOG
Professor
Department of Obstetrics
and Gynecology
Gandhi Medical College
Bhopal, Madhya Pradesh, India

Mohan A Gadam
MBBS MD FCPS DGO DFP FICS FICOG
Senior Consultant
Nanavati Max Super Specialty Hospital
BSES/MG Hospital and
Surya Hospital, Maharashtra
Director
Eva Medicare, Fertility and
Endoscopy Centre
Mumbai and Thane, Maharashtra, India
Program Director
Indu Jain Fertility Centre/Bhagwan
Mahavir Hospital
Pali, Rajasthan, India
Past Head
Dr RN Cooper Hospital, Mumbai
Past Associate Professor, LTMMC
Mumbai, Maharashtra, India

Mukesh Rathi
MBBS MD DNB FCPS DGO FICMCH
Director
Department of Obstetrics
and Gynecology
Laxminarayan Memorial Hospital
Akola, Maharashtra, India

Narendra Gajjar
MBBS MD DG
Consultant
Department of Obstetrics
and Gynecology
Ashirwad Hospital and
Akash IVF Centre
Navsari and Chikhali, Gujarat, India

Nidhi Sharma Chauhann MBBS MS
Consultant Gynecologist
Department of Obstetrics
and Gynecology
Saifee Hospital
Mumbai, Maharashtra, India

Nikita Gadam MBBS MD DNBE FRM
Consultant, BSES/MG Hospital, Mumbai
Director, Eva Medicare, Fertility
and Endoscopy Centre
Mumbai and Thane, Maharashtra, India
Visiting Consultant, Indu Jain Fertility
Centre/Bhagwan Mahavir Hospital
Sumerpur, Rajasthan, India

Nilakshi Phukan Kumar MBBS MD
Consultant
Department of Obstetrics
and Gynecology
Down Town Hospital
Guwahati, Assam, India

Pankaj Sarode MBBS MD FICS
Consultant
Department of Obstetrics
and Gynecology
Cradle Maternity and Women Care
Pune, Maharashtra, India

Punam Dixit
MBBS (Hons) MS MRCOG (UK) FRCOG (UK)
Consultant
Department of Obstetrics
and Gynecology
Punam Surgical and Maternity Hospital
Patna, Bihar, India

Rajshree Dayanand Katke
MD (Obs & Gyne) FICOG FMAS
Professor and Head
Department of Obstetrics
and Gynecology
St George Hospital
Mumbai, Maharashtra, India

Ramkrishna Purohit MBBS MD FICOG
Director
Department of Obstetrics
and Gynecology
Purohit General Hospital
Bargarh, Odisha, India

Richa Narkhede MBBS MD
Assistant Professor
Department of Obstetrics
and Gynecology
Sri Aurobindo Institute of
Medical Sciences
Indore, Madhya Pradesh, India

RM Saraogi MBBS MD DGO FCPS
Director
Department of Obstetrics
and Gynecology
Saraogi Group of Hospitals, Mumbai
Senior Consultant
Department of Obstetrics
and Gynecology
Nanavati Hospital
Mumbai, Maharashtra, India

Sandhya Panigrahi
FICOG MICOG FICMCH FAIOG FCGP
Senior Consultant
Gayatri Clinic
Ganjam, Odisha, India

Sonal Bathla MBBS MD
Director and Head
Department of Obstetrics
and Gynecology
Yatharth Superspecialty Hospital
New Delhi, India

Sonam Kataria MBBS MS DNB
Consultant
Department of Obstetrics
and Gynecology
RMS Multispeciality Hospital
Mumbai, Maharashtra, India

Suman Sinha
MBBS DGO FICOG FIAOG FIAMS
Senior Consultant
Department of Obstetrics
and Gynecology
Global Synergy Hospital
Ranchi, Jharkhand, India

Uma Rani Swain MBBS MD
Senior Director
Department of Obstetrics
and Gynecology
BLK-Max Super Specialty Hospital
New Delhi, India

Preface

The updated *Manual on Shirish Sheth: Vaginal Surgery* by FOGSI, features 14 comprehensive chapters that embodies the entire spectrum of vaginal surgeries. It has been presented in a very crisp and concise manner with the sole purpose of imparting basics and fundamental knowledge to enhance the surgical skills of the practicing doctors and students. The authors have dedicated countless hours to meticulously compiling the chapters. We are immensely thankful to them.

We are equally obliged and grateful to our Dr Sunita Tandulwadkar (President, FOGSI), Dr Bhaskar Pal (President-Elect FOGSI), Dr Suvarna Khadilkar (Secretary General, FOGSI), Dr Ashok Kumar (Organizing Chairperson, AICOG), Dr Neerja Bhatla (Scientific Chairperson, AICOG), Dr K Aparna Sharma and Dr Madhavi M Gupta (Organizing Secretary, AICOG) for believing in us and giving us the opportunity. We are indebted to them for their unwavering support and guidance.

Our sincere thanks to Shri Jitendar P Vij (Group Chairman) and Mr Ankit Vij (Managing Director) of M/s Jaypee Brothers Medical Publishers (P) Ltd, New Delhi, India for their support, encouragement and logistic. We express our special thanks to the entire production team of M/s Jaypee Brothers Medical Publishers (P) Ltd especially, Mr Priyansh Saxena (Development Editor) and Nikita Chauhan for their hard work, Professionalism and for helping us throughout the journey of this publication.

May this manual be a guiding light to serve as an invaluable resource in understanding the intricacies of vaginal surgeries for our practitioners and academicians.

Knowledge is Power, Never Stop Learning

Happy Learning to our readers.

***Editors:* Rajendra Saraogi, Suman Sinha, Meenakshi, Nishi Makhija**

Contents

1 CHAPTER

Advancing NDVH Practices in LSCS: Trends, Challenges, and Opportunities

Sonal Bathla, Richa Narkhede

INTRODUCTION

Cesarean deliveries have increased significantly in last 15 years by about 54% in US from 1996 to 2007. Annually, over 18 million cesarean births are documented worldwide, accounting for roughly 19.1% of all deliveries. Rate of vaginal birth after cesarean delivery too has decreased significantly from 28 to 8% in the said period. This contributes significantly to an increasing burden of scarred uteri. Now because of increased rate of cesarean section, the number of women requesting hysterectomies postcesarean section is also increasing. Historically, a prior cesarean was considered a relative contraindication to vaginal hysterectomy due to concerns as utero-vesical adhesions and the risk of unintended cystostomy. But now with advancing surgical skills, even prior multiple cesarean is no longer considered a contraindication.

ADVANTAGES OF NDVH OVER LAP HYSTERECTOMY IN PREVIOUS CESAREAN SECTION

Nondescent vaginal hysterectomy is associated with no scar, not even the scar of the port. The removal of the uterus is undertaken through the natural orifice. This surgery is associated with less operative time, less intraoperative bleeding, less postoperative morbidity and early discharge from the hospital. There is no extra setup cost, only conventional instruments are required. No specially trained assistant is required and is not associated with the risk of incisional hernia. The criteria laid down for case selection, however, should be appropriately met.

INCLUSION CRITERIA FOR NDVH IN PREVIOUS CS

The inclusion criteria advocate that the size of the uterus should not be >14 weeks. Adnexal pathology should be ruled out by preoperative ultrasonography, mobility of the uterus should not be restricted and hysterectomy should be planned for benign causes or very early stage of malignancy. The Sheth's sign suggesting adhesions between uterus and anterior abdominal wall should be negative in patient planned for NDVH.

TABLE 1: Indications, relative contraindications and contraindications for NDVH.

Indications	*Relative contraindication*	*Contraindication*
Dysfunctional uterine bleeding	Uterus >14 weeks size	Absence of free mobility
Fibroid	Shallow fornices	Uterus size >20 weeks/ volume >400 cc
Abnormal uterine bleeding	Previous multiple scars	Frozen pelvis
Adenomyosis	Bladder/rectum reaching the tip of cervix	Diseases of bowel, omentum
Chronic pelvic pain	Short cervix	Ovarian, endometrial, cervical Ca
Postmenopausal bleeding	Limited vaginal space	Severe endometriosis
Pyometra	Multiple huge fibroids	Cervical amputation
Cervical dysplasia/polyp	Endometriosis	Inaccessible cervix
Benign adnexal pathology		Vesicovaginal fistula repair
Carcinoma in situ of cervix		Invasive cancer of cervix
Endometrial ca		

Source: Ray A, Pant L, Magon N. Deciding the route for hysterectomy: Indian triage system. J Obstet Gynaecol India. 2015;65(1):39-44.

Exclusion Criteria for NDVH in Previous CS

NDVH in patient with previous CS should be avoided if the size of the uterus is >14 weeks, cervix is inaccessible and there is a restricted mobility of the uterus and the cervix. Any complicated adnexal pathology or genital malignancy must be ruled out.

CLINICAL ASSESSMENT FOR A SUCCESSFUL VAGINAL SURGERY

The patient is laid down in dorsal position after she empties her bladder. After a thorough systemic examination, the abdomen is inspected for any mass or scar of a previous surgery. An assessment of vaginal space is undertaken. Vaginal inaccessibility is defined as intertuberous diameter <9 cm, a suprapubic angle <90 degrees and a vagina <2 finger widths in caliber. The cervix should not be pulled up and fixed. Uterine volume, transverse diameter of uterus should be assessed on ultrasonography. Uterus, which is expanded more in transverse diameter is difficult to deliver. Sheth's cervico-fundal sign to anticipate adhesions with anterior abdominal wall is elicited. Stretched posterior vaginal wall pulled upwards in its upper half, inability to visualize cervix or cervix placed almost behind the public symphysis is difficult to deliver vaginally.

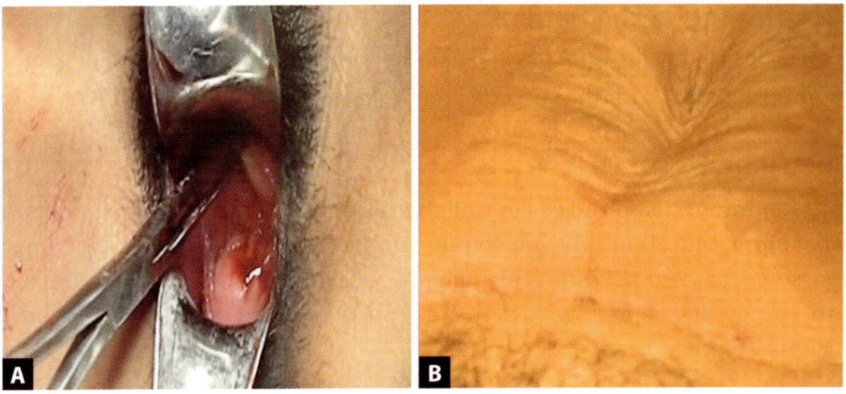

Figs. 1A and B: Pulled up cervix, dimpling sign on examination.
Courtesy: Narkhede Richa, OPD examination procedure. Photograph in author's possession.

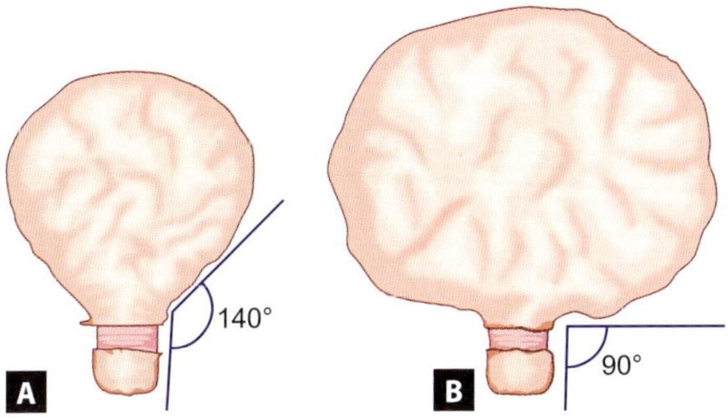

Figs. 2A and B: Fibroids which pose a difficulty for NDVH.
Source: Sheth SS, Paghdiwalla KP, Hajari AR. Vaginal route: a gynaecological route for much more than hysterectomy. Best Prac Res Clin Obstet Gynaecol. 2011;25(2):115-32.

Traction on cervix creating dimple on the lower abdominal wall, rules out the vaginal approach for hysterectomy **(Figs. 1A and B)**.

Fibroids Which Pose a Difficulty for NDVH

Fibroids at utero cervical junction decreasing the angle to <90°, fundal fibroids with diameter >10 cm, lateral extension of the fibroids to broad ligament, degenerated fibroids in a big uterus, fibroids causing gross asymmetry of uterus or cervical fibroids are difficult to deliver vaginally, however the outcome is influenced more by the surgical skill **(Fig. 2A and B)**.

Consent and Documentation

Patient and her relatives must be counseled regarding the approach to hysterectomy, possibility of conversion, risk of bladder injury and risk of prolonged catheterization. The decision for the conservation of tubes and ovaries must be discussed and documented. Preoperative anesthesia clearance should be taken after appropriate investigations.

Positioning of the Patient

Dorsal lithotomy position flexing the thighs towards the abdomen creates an appropriate space for the surgeon and her assistants **(Figs. 3A and B)**.

Instruments for NDVH

The common, cheap and easily available instruments for NDVH include sim's speculum, vulsellum uterine sound, surgical knife, hysterectomy clamps, scissors, Vicryl no 1 suture, artery forceps, allis forceps and Deaver's retractor. An energy device as LigaSure may be used in place of the hysterectomy clamps **(Fig. 4)**.

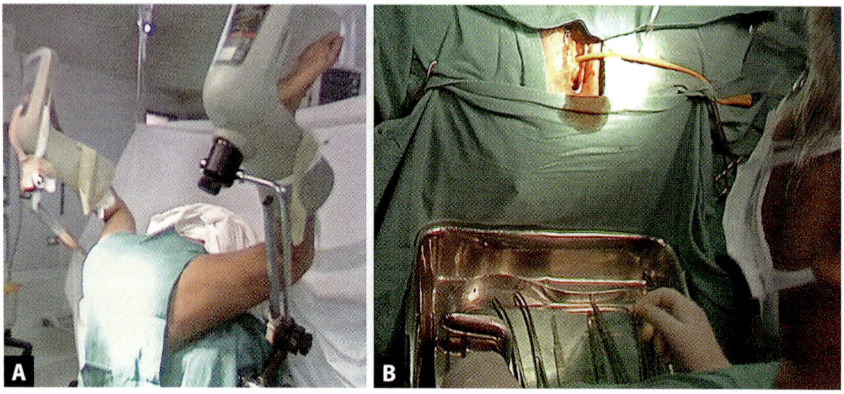

Figs. 3A and B: Positioning of the patient and relative position of surgeon, tray, and the patient.
Courtesy: Bathla, Sonal. NVDH procedure, 2025. Photograph in author's possession.

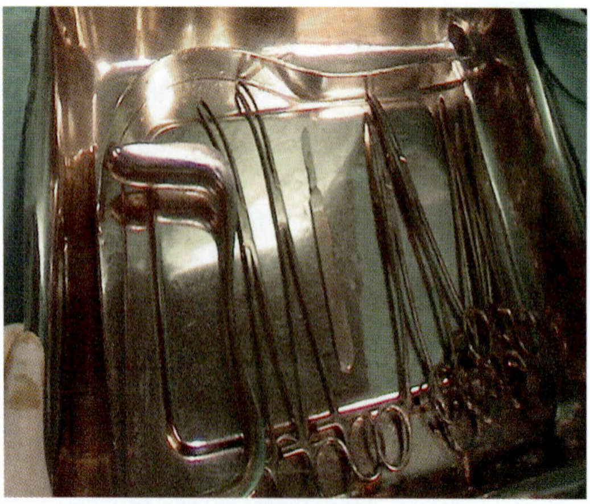

Fig. 4: Instruments.
Courtesy: Bathla S. NVDH procedure, 2025. Photograph in author's possession.

PROCEDURE FOR NDVH IN PREVIOUS CESAREAN SECTION

The anterior and posterior lip of the cervix are held with vulsellum and the posterior vaginal wall is retracted with sim's speculum. A solution of 200 mL of normal saline with one ampoule of adrenaline, i.e., 1:200,000 solution is infiltrated. The infiltration helps in reaching the exact plane between bladder and the uterus and adrenaline helps in maintaining hemostasis by vasoconstriction **(Fig. 5)**.

A circular incision is given around the cervix and the posterior pouch is opened by sharp dissection. The pubo-vesico-cervical ligament is dissected and the bladder is mobilized upward. Bilateral Mackenrodt's ligaments are clamped cut and ligated.

At the site of the previous scar, the bladder is dissected by a lateral window approach. The concept is that the bladder is adherent in the central three fifth and not in the lateral one fifth. So, dissect in the lateral one fifth on either side and enter into a surgical window between uterocervical surface posteriorly and the bladder anteriorly, i.e.; the Sheth's utero cervical broad ligament space. The anterior wall of this space is formed by the undersurface of the lowermost portion of bladder, the lateral wall by the anterior leaf of broad ligament, posterior wall is formed medially by uterocervical surface space and laterally by the posterior leaf of the broad ligament.

Bilateral uterine arteries are clamped, cut and ligated after opening the anterior pouch. Uterine debulking for retrieval is carried out by cervical amputation, bisection, myomectomy, Pryor's technique, wedge morcellation and Lash's intramyometrial coring.

The cornual structures are clamped, cut and ligated. One may consider prophylactic salpingectomy at this step if ovaries are conserved. If decision of oophorectomy is taken then the round ligament is ligated first, followed by

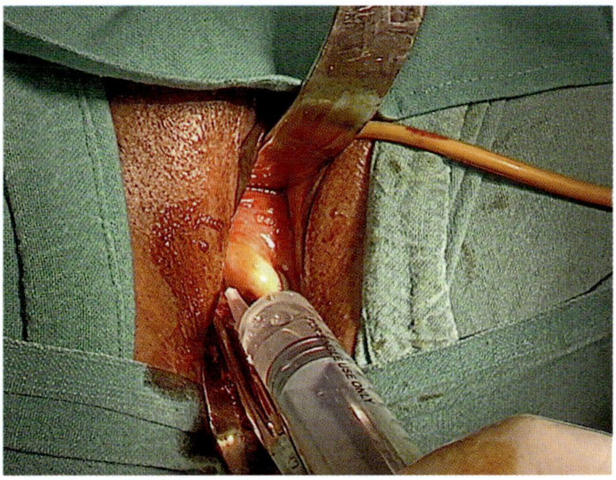

Fig. 5: Saline infiltration for better dissection.
Courtesy: Bathla S. NVDH procedure, 2025. Photograph in author's possession.

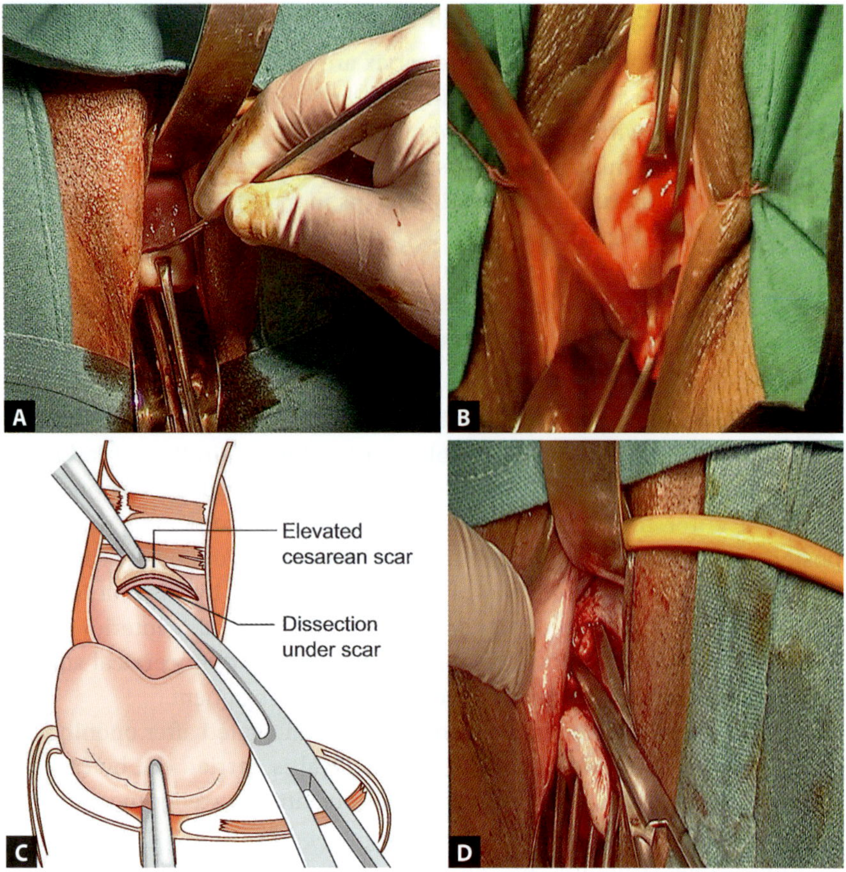

Figs. 6A to D: Circular incision, opening of pouch of Douglas, and pubo-vesico-cervical ligament dissection.
Courtesy: Bathla, Sonal. NVDH procedure, 2025. Photograph in author's possession.

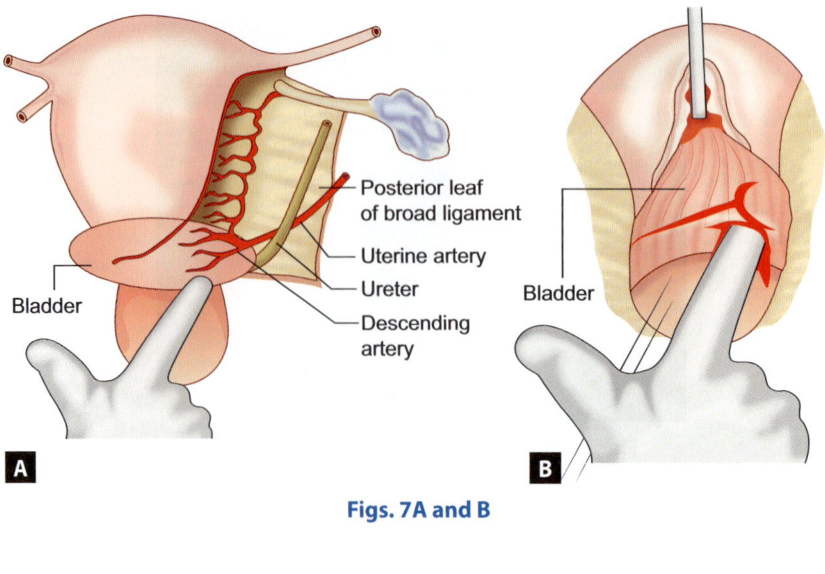

Figs. 7A and B

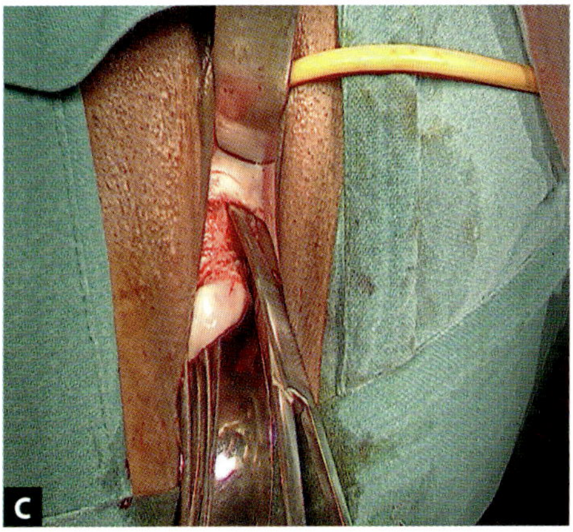

Fig. 7C

Figs. 7A to C: Showing sharp dissection through the lateral window.
Source: Sheth SS, Paghdiwalla KP, Hajari AR. Vaginal route: A gynaecological route for much more than hysterectomy. Best Pract Res Clin Obstet Gynaecol. 2011;25(2):115-32.

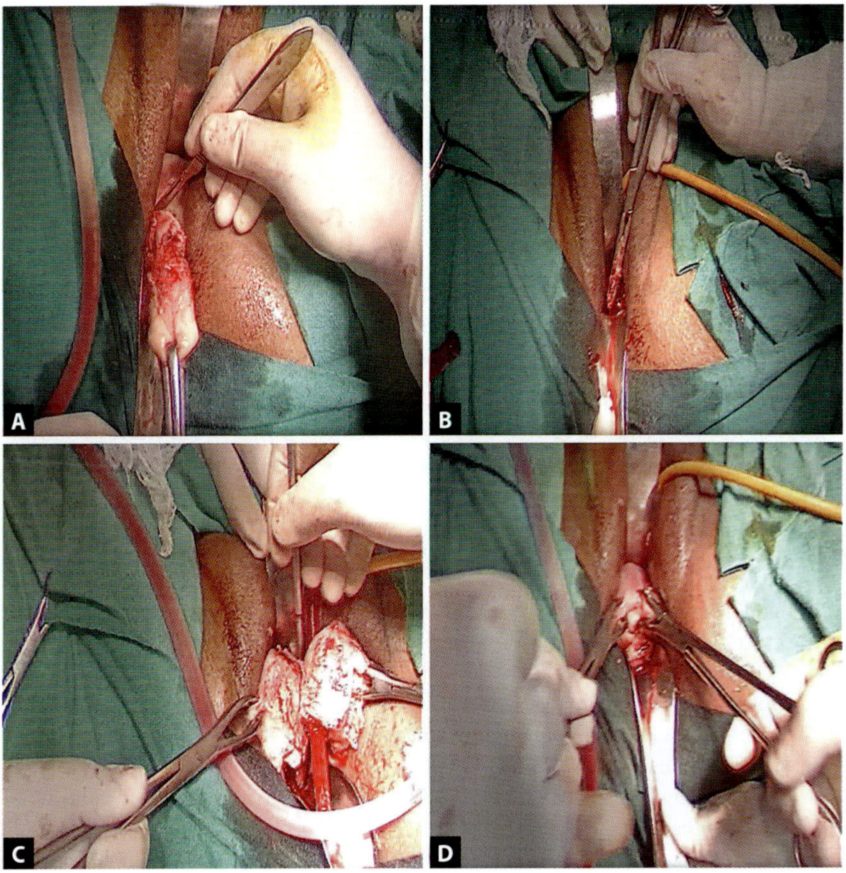

Figs. 8A to D: Morcellation.
Courtesy: Bathla, Sonal. NVDH procedure, 2025. Photograph in author's possession.

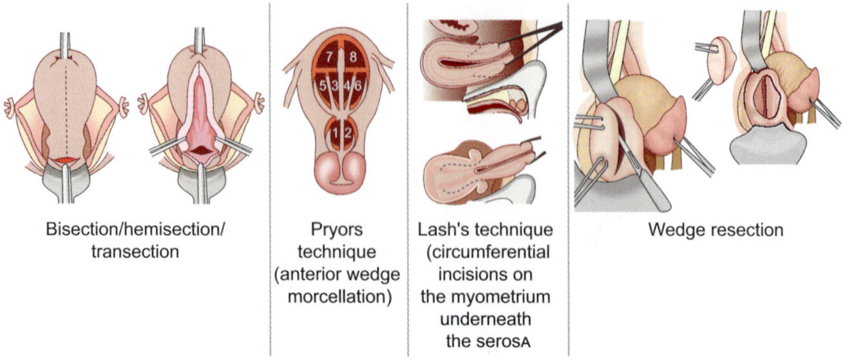

Fig. 9: Diagrammatic representation of morcellation.
Source: Marco A PII, Marco A PIII. Uterine Debulking at Vaginal Hysterectomy. In: Shirish S (Ed). Vaginal Hysterectomy. New Delhi: Jaypee Brothers Medical Publishers; 2014.

the infundibulopelvic ligament. Culdoplasty is undertaken to prevent vault prolapse. The Mackenrodt and the uterosacral ligaments help in suspending the angles of the vault to the lateral pelvic wall. Vault is closed by interrupted interlocking sutures starting from both the angles after ensuring complete hemostasis and swab count. A LigaSure may alternatively be used for all the pedicles.

Postoperatively patient may be catheterized for one day, kept on broad spectrum antibiotics and vaginal packing is optional.

CONCLUSION

Vaginal hysterectomy for benign indications associated with previous cesarean section may be accomplished safely in the absence of fixed adhesions of the uterine corpus to anterior abdominal wall. The lateral window approach and hydro dissection may avoid unintended bladder injury in the presence of dense utero vesical adhesions. Every patient should be tried for vaginal route hysterectomy unless contraindicated. It is safe, comfortable and cost effective.

SUGGESTED READING

1. Balakrishnan D, Dibyajyoti G. A comparison between non descent vaginal hysterectomy and total abdominal hysterectomy. J Clin Diagn Res. 2016;10(1):11-4.
2. Duong TH, Patterson TM. Lower urinary tract injuries during hysterectomy in women with a history of two or more cesarean deliveries: a secondary analysis Int Urogynaecol J. 2014;25(8):1037-40.
3. El-Shawarby SA, Salim R, Lavery S. Uterine adherence to anterior abdominal wall after caesarean section. BJOG. 2011;118:1133.
4. Lafay Pillet MC, Leonard F, Chopin N. Incidence and risk factors of bladder injuries during laproscopic hysterectomy indicated for benign uterine

pathologies: a14.5 years experience in a continuous series of 1501 procedures. Hum Reprod. 2009;24:842.
5. Nalini N, Bijeta, Kumari S. Previous LSCS: no more contraindication for non descent vaginal hysterectomy. Int J Contemporary Med Res. 2018;5(8):H1-H4.
6. Purohit RK, Sharma JP, Singh S, Giri DK. Vaginal hysterectomy by electrosurgery for benign indications associated with previous cesarean section. J Gynaecol Surg. 2013;29(1):7-12.
7. Rooney CM, Crawford AT, Vassallo BJ. Is previous cesarean section a risk for incidental cystotomy at the time of hysterectomy? A case-controlled study. Am J Obstet Gynecol. 2005;193:2041.
8. Sheth S, Shah NM, Varaiya D. A sonographic and clinical sign to detect specific adhesions following cesarean section. J Gynecol Surg. 2008;24:27.
9. Sheth SS, Goyal MV, Shah N. Uterocervical displacement following adhesions after cesarean section. J Gynecol Surg. 1997;13:143.
10. Sheth SS. Uterocervical broad ligament space. In: Radhika AG (ed). Non descent vaginal hysterectomy 2013.

2 CHAPTER

Adnexectomy at Vaginal Hysterectomy

Elizabeth Jacob, Ganpat Sawant

INTRODUCTION

Vaginal adnexectomy refers to the surgical removal of the ovaries (oophorectomy) and/or fallopian tubes (salpingectomy), or the complete adnexal structures (salpingo-oophorectomy) via the vaginal route. The vaginal approach offers distinct advantages including reduced postoperative pain, faster recovery, better cosmesis with absence of abdominal scars, and lower overall morbidity compared to abdominal or laparoscopic routes.

The need to perform oophorectomy should not be considered a contraindication to vaginal hysterectomy. It is possible to perform oophorectomy at the time of vaginal hysterectomy in >90% of properly selected cases. Good vaginal retraction, appropriate instrumentation, adequate lighting and enthusiastic assistants are the key to successful outcome while performing vaginal adnexectomy.

INDICATIONS (TABLE 1)

- Prophylactic salpingectomy
- Prophylactic oophorectomy
- Removal of tubo-ovarian pathology

Vaginal oophorectomy was successful in 94% of the patients. Factors influencing the success include obesity, nulliparity, decreased vaginal access and space, lack of uterine descent, increased uterine size and tubo-ovarian disease.

TABLE 1: Indications for vaginal adnexectomy.

Category	*Specific indications*
Benign ovarian pathology	• Simple ovarian cysts (functional, serous cystadenoma) • Benign ovarian tumors (mature cystic teratoma) • Paraovarian cysts
Prophylactic/risk-reducing	• BSO in postmenopausal women at hysterectomy • BRCA1/BRCA2 mutation carriers (age 35–45 years) • Lynch syndrome patients • Strong family history of ovarian/breast cancer • Opportunistic salpingectomy for cancer prevention

CONTRAINDICATIONS (TABLE 2)

Laparoscopic assistance and V notes can help surpass many of the contraindications for performing vaginal adnexectomy.

SURGICAL TECHNIQUES

Conventional Vaginal Adnexectomy—Surgical Steps

After vaginal hysterectomy:

- *Ovarian delivery:* Gentle traction on round ligament/ovarian ligament
- *IP ligament identification:* Trace ovary laterally to ovarian vessels and ensure that it's free of adhesions
- *Ureteral safety:* Confirm ureter is medial and inferior to infundibulopelvic ligament
- *IP ligament clamping:* Apply curved Heaney/specialized clamp **(Fig. 1)**

TABLE 2: Contraindications to vaginal adnexectomy.

Type	*Contraindications*
Absolute	• Suspected or confirmed ovarian malignancy requiring staging • Large adnexal masses (>10 cm) with high malignancy risk • Dense pelvic adhesions obliterating pouch of Douglas • Severe PID with tubo-ovarian abscess
Relative	• Nulliparity with narrow vaginal access • Previous multiple pelvic surgeries • Moderate endometriosis with expected adhesions • Morbid obesity (BMI >35 kg/m^2) • Large ovarian masses (6–10 cm)

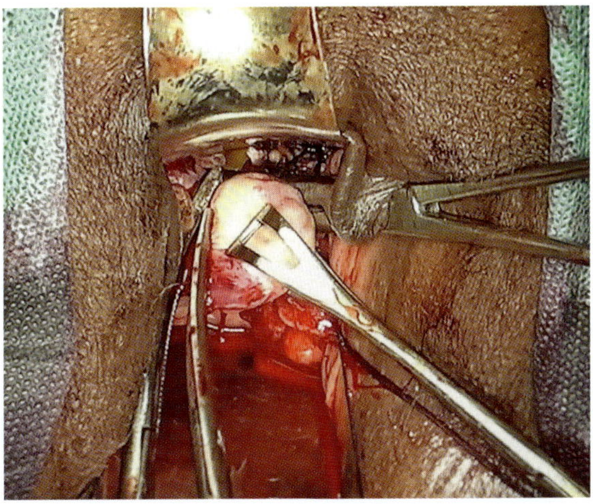

Fig. 1: Clamping infundibulopelvic ligament.

- *Division and ligation:* Divide between clamps, transfixion suture (0/1-0 vicryl)
- Hemostasis verification
- *Specimen removal:* Extract intact or in specimen bag

Alternative Techniques

Different modifications have been proposed to circumvent the difficulty to access the ovaries vaginally.

Roeder's Loop

Access to ovaries by Roeder's loop used in laparoscopic surgery to get around the ovary has been used especially in postmenopausal atrophic laterally placed ovaries when access to applying clamps may be difficult.

Sheth's Special Adnexa Clamp

Vaginal oophorectomy was successful in 94% of the patients in a series of 740 patients using the specialized Sheth's clamp. Sheth's adnexa clamp for the IP ligament/mesovarium has a favorable curve beginning at 1 cm from the tip for a distance of 2 cm.

Paily's Vaginal Oophorectomy Clamp

The Paily's Vaginal Oophorectomy Clamp's reversed blade design allows direct and secure grasping of the infundibulopelvic ligament as there is no intervening tissue near the joint, reducing the risk of slippage. A distinctive feature is the reversed blade at the cranial end, bent backward for 2 cm **(Fig. 2)**. This reversed design allows for the direct and secure grasping of the infundibulopelvic ligament, ensuring no intervening tissue near the joint. It provides a secure grip on the ligament and its vessels, reducing the risk of slippage and subsequent hematoma formation.

Both endoloop sutures or bipolar electrosurgery have also been tried to successfully perform vaginal adnexectomy. Prior adnexal surgery may be a confounding factor for the successful completion of adnexectomy & women with the same should be counselled appropriately.

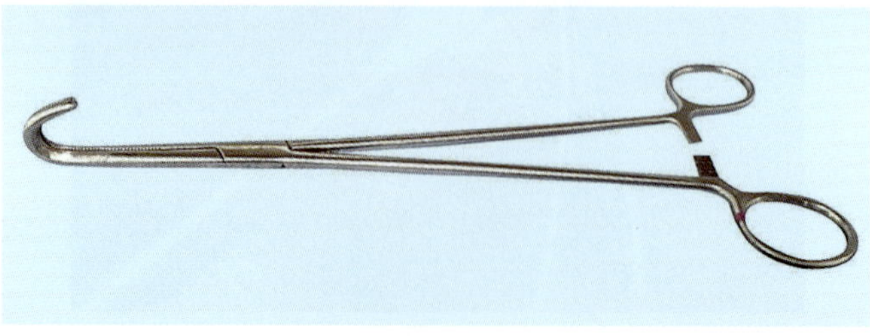

Fig. 2: Paily's vaginal oophorectomy reverse angle clamp.

TROUBLE SHOOTING AT VAGINAL ADNEXECTOMY

- Visibility and accessibility of ovaries are the most determining factors
- Side which has easy access to ovaries should be approached first
- While clamping fundal pedicles it is better that the round ligament is taken separately to prevent bunching of fundal pedicles
- Ovary should be held by Babcock to ensure lifting up the infundibulopelvic ligament from the lateral pelvic wall to avoid injury to ureter
- Avoid undue traction on the ovary
- Confirm tube and ovary are completely free of adhesions before applying clamps.

COMPLICATIONS AND MANAGEMENT

- *Hemorrhage from IP ligament:*
  - *Prevention:* Secure clamping technique, secure ligature
  - *Management:* Apply pressure, re-clamp proximally after proper exposure, secure ligature
  - *If uncontrolled:* Convert to laparoscopy/laparotomy for vascular control
- *Ureteral injury:*
  - *Prevention:* Proper anatomical knowledge of ureter course, maintain adequate distance from IP ligament, ensure ovary free of adhesions prior to applying the clamp
  - *Management:* If injury recognized intraoperatively—immediate urological consultation, repair over stent
- *Bowel injury:*
  - *Prevention:* Identify the risk factors (Adhesions due to previous surgeries, endometriosis, PID), proper case selection, laparoscopic assistance if adhesions suspected
  - *Management:* Small serosal injury—primary repair; full-thickness injury—surgical/colorectal consultation

CONVERSION TO LAPAROSCOPY/LAPAROTOMY

Proper informed consent and appropriate counselling should be done preoperatively especially in patients with benign adnexal masses, previous surgeries and endometriosis. In adnexal masses, proper selection of cases to ensure the benign nature of the mass and to select cases free of adhesions, mobile and close to POD for vaginal removal will be paramount to successful outcome.

Conversion to laparoscopy/laparotomy should be undertaken if there is:

- Uncontrolled bleeding
- Slippage of pedicles
- Incompleteness

Flowchart 1: Oophorectomy at VH.

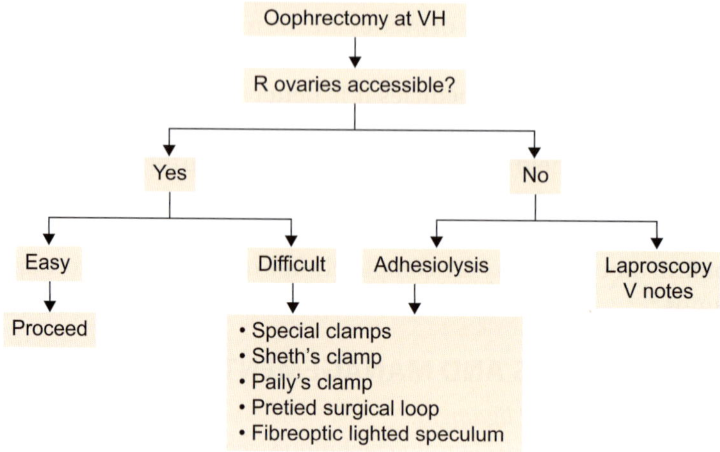

- Inability to access adnexa
- Suspected malignancy
- Dense adhesions
- Major organ injury

It should not be thought of as a failure, rather it should be considered as an appropriate surgical judgment for ensuring patient safety **(Flowchart 1)**.

KEY PRACTICE POINTS

- Vaginal adnexectomy is a safe, effective and minimally invasive approach for benign adnexal pathology. It should be the preferred approach when technically feasible.
- Careful preoperative assessment including imaging (transvaginal ultrasound), tumor markers, and RMI calculation is crucial to exclude malignancy and ensure appropriate case selection.
- Visibility and accessibility of ovaries are the most determining factors while performing vaginal adnexectomy
- Key surgical principles include: meticulous identification of infundibulopelvic ligament, ensuring ureteral safety, secure vascular pedicle ligation ,ensuring the ovary is free of adhesions prior to applying the clamp and taking aid of the specialized clamps in difficult cases.
- Conversion to laparoscopy or laparotomy represents appropriate surgical judgment and not failure. It should be resorted to in cases of uncontrolled hemorrhage, inability to access adnexa, suspected malignancy, or major organ injury.
- vNOTES combines advantages of vaginal surgery (no abdominal scars, faster recovery) with laparoscopic visualization, offering enhanced surgical precision with comparable or superior outcomes to conventional laparoscopy and should be considered in cases of difficulty via the conventional vaginal route.
- Good vaginal retraction, appropriate instrumentation, adequate lighting, and enthusiastic assistants are the key to successful outcome while performing vaginal adnexectomy along with the strong determination of the surgeon and great teamwork.

SUGGESTED READING

1. Antosh DD, High R, Brown HW, Oliphant SS, Abed H, Philip N, et al. Feasibility of prophylactic salpingectomy during vaginal hysterectomy. Am J Obstet Gynecol. 2017;217(5):605.e1–605.e5.
2. Camanni M, Mistrangelo E, Febo G, Ferrero B, Deltetto F. Prophylactic bilateral oophorectomy during vaginal hysterectomy for benign pathology. Arch Gynecol Obstet. 2009;280(1):87-90.
3. Davies A, O'Connor H, Magos AL. A prospective study to evaluate oophorectomy at the time of vaginal hysterectomy. Br J Obstet Gynaecol. 1996;103(9):915-20.
4. Paily VP, Raj Girijadevi R, K Shefeek S. Salpingo-Oophorectomy during non-descent vaginal hysterectomy using the paily vaginal oophorectomy clamp. J Obstet Gynaecol Can. 2024;46(3):102281.
5. Sheth SS. The place of oophorectomy at vaginal hysterectomy. J Obstet Gynaecol. 1991;98(7):662-6.

3 CHAPTER

Innovations in Vaginal Surgery

Suman Sinha, Punam Dixit

INTRODUCTION AND OBJECTIVE

The field of vaginal surgery has evolved beyond its traditional boundaries, integrating novel concepts and refined techniques that have significantly broadened its clinical applications. With a growing emphasis on minimally invasive approaches, the vaginal route offers distinct advantages in terms of reduced postoperative morbidity, shorter hospital stays, and greater patient satisfaction, while maintaining surgical precision and therapeutic efficacy.

Recent innovations have revitalized interest in vaginal access for complex gynecological procedures such as vaginal myomectomy, ovarian cystectomy via the vaginal route, cervical cerclage, Vnotes combines traditional vaginal surgery with endoscopic assistance and selective clamping of the uterine arteries. These advancements exemplify the progressive adaptation of conventional principles to meet modern surgical goals, emphasizing organ preservation, reduced invasiveness, and enhanced reproductive outcomes.

This article aims to review the current innovations and technical progress in these areas, outlining their indications, operative nuances, and outcomes. A deeper understanding of these developments is essential to optimize patient selection, improve training in vaginal surgery, and integrate these techniques into contemporary gynecological practice.

VAGINAL MYOMECTOMY: TECHNIQUE AND CASE SELECTION

Myomectomy via the vaginal route, though less commonly performed, represents an excellent option in carefully selected patients. The procedure was first described by Magos et al. in 1994. Appropriate case selection and thorough preoperative evaluation are critical for optimal outcomes. Parous women with easily accessible fibroids are ideal candidates. Imaging and fibroid mapping should be performed to determine the exact location and size. Posterior wall fibroids can be accessed and removed via a posterior colpotomy incision. Prolapsed submucous and small intracervical fibroids can also be removed efficiently. The procedure involves injecting dilute vasopressin to control blood loss, enucleating the myoma, closing dead space with interrupted sutures, and securing hemostasis prior to closing the colpotomy incision.

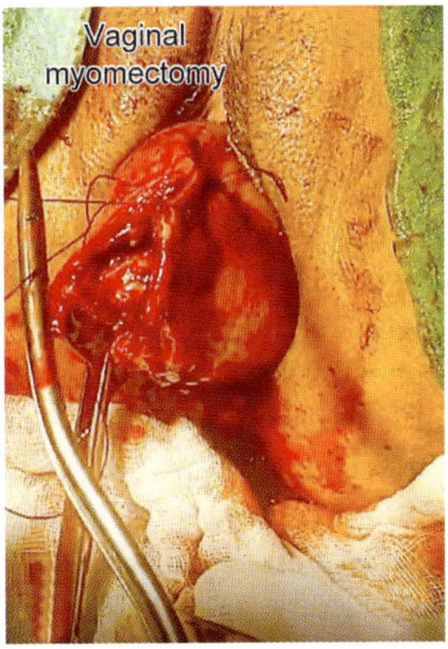

Fig. 1: Removal of post wall fibroids.

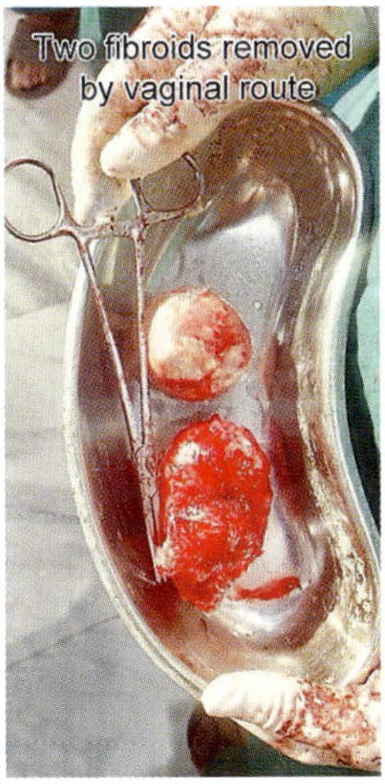

Fig. 2: Two fibroids removed (5 × 6) cms.

CERVICAL FIBROIDS: SPECIAL CONSIDERATIONS

Cervical fibroids comprise 0.6–7.7% of all leiomyomas, presenting unique challenges for laparoscopic or open approaches. Vaginal intracapsular myomectomy (CIME) has been evaluated in a case series of 32 patients, indicating feasibility and efficiency. Large anterior cervical fibroids have also been successfully removed vaginally, with various reports supporting the vaginal route in selected cases.

VAGINAL OVARIAN CYSTECTOMY: INDICATIONS AND METHOD

Vaginal ovarian cystectomy is an innovative approach for benign ovarian cysts, ideally in the absence of adhesions or endometriosis. Preoperative assessment should use the International Ovarian Tumor Analysis (IOTA) criteria. The cyst can be exteriorized or aspirated, and after removal, the ovary is returned to the peritoneal cavity, with the incision closed. Clinical studies report shorter operative time, lower postoperative pain, and higher patient satisfaction compared to abdominal or laparoscopic methods. Intraoperative ultrasound enhances surgical safety and accuracy.

Modified Shirodkar Cerclage Technique

It is one of the most important interventions to prevent premature birth. Compared with the Macdonald's and original Shirodkar's technique, there is less trauma and blood loss. The Shirodkar technique, enables high placement of the suture in the poor anatomical situation of the cervix such as funneling at the internal os, incompetent cervix, deeply lacerated cervix or extremely short cervix.

Technique

A transverse incision of about 1.5 cm is made through the anterior vaginal mucosa at its junction with the cervix. Similar transverse incision is made at the posterior vaginal mucosa at junction with the cervix.

The bladder is pushed away from the cervix anteriorly after a transverse incision on the vaginal wall and pushed upward to expose the area of the internal os, to enable high placement of the cerclage. A curved round needle 35 mm in length and 1.6 mm in diameter, with Teflon tape/Marceline/Black silk is passed through the anterior para cervical tissue. The same procedure is done at the posterior end and the knot is tied anteriorly. A continuous absorbable ligature closes the incision. Three changes were adopted in the modified Shirodkar technique: (1) To hold and compress the paracervical tissue atraumatic forceps was used. (2) The location of the knot is made at anterior fornix makes it easier to remove. (3) A Silk thread is passed through the cerclage tape assisting in easier removal of the tape by pulling the silk thread.

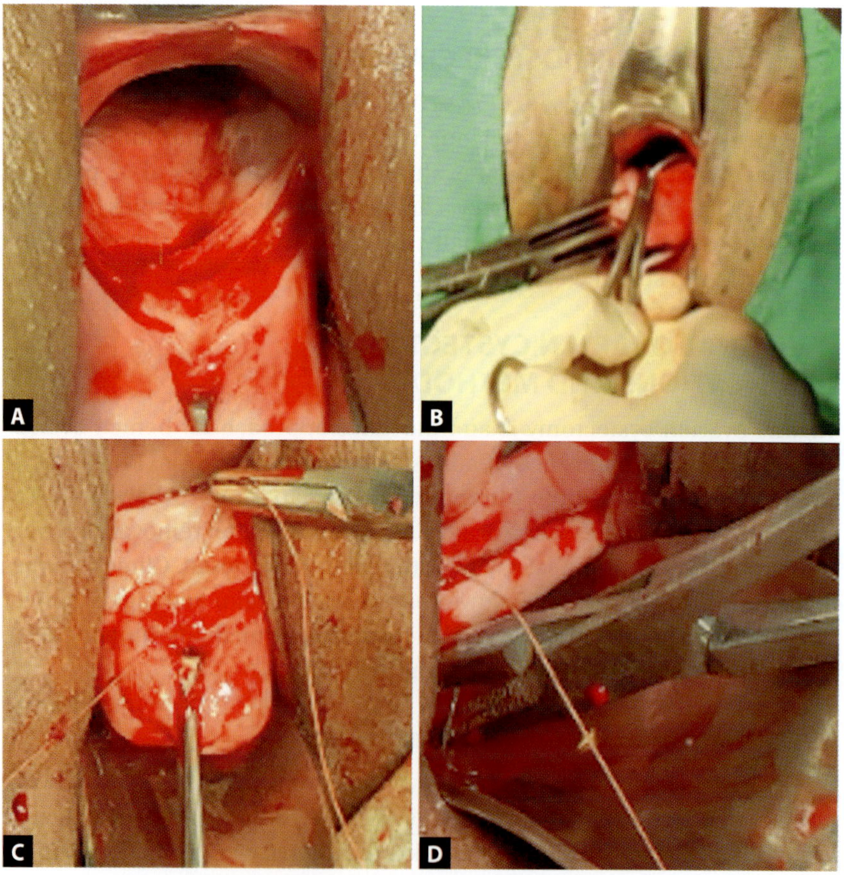

Figs. 3A to D: (A) Bladder mobilized; (B) Marceline tape being passed; (C) Closure of ant Colpotomy; (D) Closure of Posterior colpotomy.

STEPS OF MODIFIED SHIRODKAR CERVICAL CERCLAGE TECHNIQUE

vNOTES

Vaginal Natural Orifice Trans luminal Endoscopic Surgery, is an advanced surgical approach that combines traditional vaginal surgery with Endoscopic tools, resulting in better cosmetic outcomes, less pain and faster recovery times.

Technique

A circular paracervical incision is given followed by dissection of the posterior vaginal pouch down to the peritoneum which is opened. The dissection allows the exposure of the uterosacral ligaments which are cut and ligated to be later attached to the vaginal vault for prevention of vault prolapse. Then the vesicouterine space is dissected till the peritoneum and the vesicouterine pouch is opened (Anterior colpotomy). The Alexis retractor is inserted in the ant pouch opening. Then the posterior part is placed. It helps to place the platform. Patient is then placed in 20° Trendelenburg and the cavity is infiltrated with 8 mm gas. Peritoneal exploration is done under vision. First the left uterine pedicle is coagulated , followed by left utero ovarian pedicle and section of the mesosalpinx. Then right uterine pedicle is coagulated followed by coagulation and cutting of right infundibulopelvic ligament and then left infundibulopelvic ligament is coagulated and cut. The uterus is then removed through the opening. The Alexis retractor and platform is removed. The vault is closed in a running suture with Vicry no1. The utero sacral ligament is reattached to the vault. The patient is discharged after 24–48 hours when she is stable and has passed urine and there is no complications.

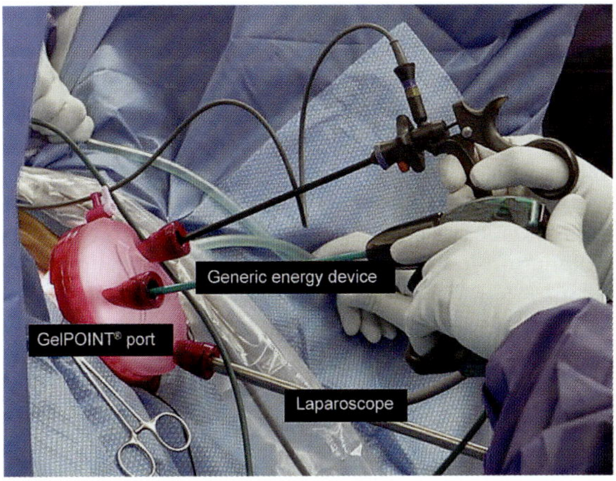

Fig. 4: Vaginal natural orifice transluminal hysterectomy.

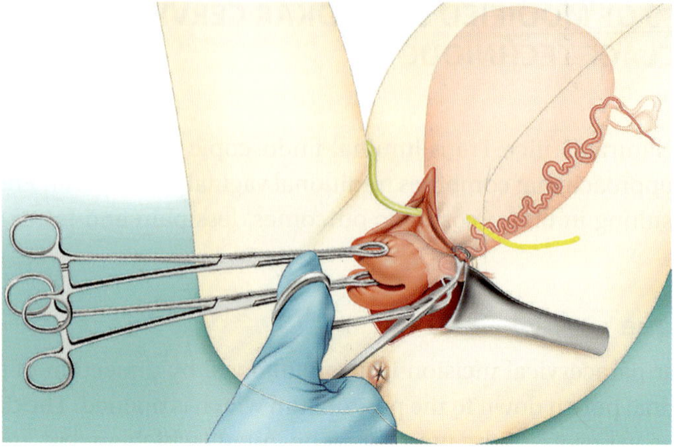

Fig. 5: Transvaginal clamping of bilateral uterine arteries.

Transvaginal Uterine Artery Clamp

A temporary intervention to stop bleeding in postpartum hemorrhage. Most of the maternal death in PPH are due to delay in management. Uterine arteries are the major contributor of blood supply to the uterus and methods to occlude these arteries can reduce perfusion effectively. In low resource setting it is a very useful device. Methods like uterine balloon tamponade do not give immediate response when every passing minute is crucial for the patient. So for quick action bilateral occlusion of uterine arteries using Trans vaginal uterine artery cervical occlusion clamp (TVUAC) is a promising device to prevent maternal morbidity and mortality in women who delivers vaginally.

KEY POINTS

- Both vaginal myomectomy and cystectomy are safe and effective with proper case selection and surgical expertise.
- These techniques yield substantial benefits, including minimally invasive access and optimized reproductive outcomes.
- Continued research and training will further enhance their adoption and standardization.
- The modified Shirodkar's technique, enables high placement of the suture in the poor anatomical situation of the cervix and thus prevents premature birth.
- Transvaginal uterine artery cervical occlusion clamp is a promising devise to control PPH in low resource settings.
- Vnotes is minimal invasive gynecological surgery done through vaginal route. Endoscopic instruments and laparoscope are inserted vaginally and surgical procedures like hysterectomy, adnexectomy can be performed under vision., offers benefits like less pain and fast recovery.

SUGGESTED READING

1. Benjamin T, Magos A. Subtotal hysterectomy and myomectomy - vaginally. Best Pract Res Clin Obstet Gynaecol. 2011;25(2):133-52.
2. Chen F, Bai F, Wang Y, Li W. Case report of a giant cervical leiomyoma. Front Med (Lausanne). 2025;11:11999.
3. Deshpandey H, Ansari AG, Choudhary PS, Madhav C. A Comparative Study of Modified Shirodkar's Cerclage and Mcdonald's Cerclage in Cervical incompetence. Indian J Obstet Gynecol Res. 2016;3(2):143-7.
4. Feyrer R, Klenk R, Wallwiener D, Isaacson KB. (2025). Gynecologic Myomectomy: Practice Essentials, History of the Procedure. [online] Available from https://emedicine.medscape.com/article/271541-overviewemedicine.medscape [Last accessed January, 2026].
5. Futcher F, George P, Habib N. V-NOTES Hysterectomy: Surgery in 10 Steps. Gynecol Minim Invasive Ther. 2024;13(1):60-1.
6. Głąb E, Nawrocka-Rutkowska J, Roszak M, Sajdak S. Clinical evaluation of transvaginal myomectomy surgery: a retrospective study of 138 cases. Ginekol Pol. 2021;92(2):152-8.
7. Joshi B, Srivastava VK, Jain PK. Cervical fibroid: a diagnostic dilemma and operative challenge. Int J Gynecol Obstet Res. 2025;12(4):454-60.
8. The journal of clinical gynaecology and obstetrics. ISSN number (1927-1271) Print and 1927-128× online, it is a quarterly, open access journal published by Elmer Press Inc. The Journal is indexed in Pubmed, Google Scholar.
9. Lerner VT, May G, Iglesia CB. Vaginal Natural Orifice Transluminal Endoscopic Surgery Revolution: The Next Frontier in Gynecologic Minimally Invasive Surgery. JSLS. 2023;27(1):e2022.00082.
10. Magos AL, Bournas N, Sinha R, O'Connor H, Richardson RE, Turnbull AC. Vaginal myomectomy. Br J Obstet Gynaecol. 1994;101(12):1092-4.
11. Nieto-Calvache AJ, Basanta N, Palacios-Jaraquemada JM, Rivera-Torres LF, Zea F. Vaginal clamping of uterine arteries: a temporary intervention to stop bleeding in postpartum hemorrhage. Am J Obstet Gynecol. 2025;233(4):341-4.
12. Paily VP, Raj G R, Sidhik A, Sudhamma A, Neelankavil JJ, Usha MG, et al. Arresting post partum haemorrhage using the novel trans vaginal uterine artery clamp Eur J Obstet Gynecol Reprod Biol. 2022;272:6-15.
13. Uchide K, UenoH, Sumitani H. Inoue Modifications to the modified Shirodkar operation. Am J Perinatol. 2000;17(8):437-9.
14. Zhang W, Sun L, Li Q, Xu Y, Wei X. Cervical fibroids: the vaginal intracapsular myomectomy with direct approach. Front Med (Lausanne). 2025;12:12345.
15. Zhu J, Xie Y, Li X, Liu Q. Intracervical intracapsular myomectomy using loop ligation. J Obstet Gynaecol Res. 2021;47(12):4381-9.

4 CHAPTER

Vaginal Hysterectomy for Uterine Fibroids: Surgical Nuances

Pankaj Sarode, Narendra Gajjar

INTRODUCTION

Vaginal hysterectomy (VH) is a minimally invasive and well-established approach for benign uterine pathologies, including uterine fibroids. It is the route of choice for all benign indications for hysterectomy. Although laparoscopic and abdominal routes are often selected for larger or multiple fibroids, VH remains feasible and advantageous when performed with refined surgical technique and appropriate patient selection.

PATIENT SELECTION

Ideal candidates include women with:

- Uterine size generally ≤16 weeks (though experienced surgeons may exceed this)
- Mobile uterus (uterus free space in the pelvis allowing specimen maneuverability).

  Clinical examination and examination under anesthesia should allow easy and ample side to side and cephalad mobility of the specimen.
- No significant pelvic adhesions or extensive prior pelvic surgery or extensive pelvic endometriosis restricting mobility of the uterus and distorting the anatomical correlations of the pelvic organs.

A few cases are contraindications for vaginal approach not due to the size but due to the location of the fibroid. One is depicted in the picture below.

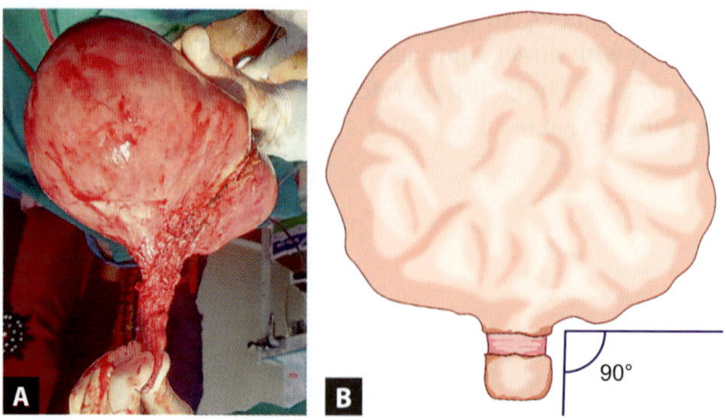

Figs. 1A and B: Acute cervico-uterine angle is a contraindication for vaginal route. *Courtesy*: Dr Pankaj Sarode. *Diagram:* Dr Shirish Seth

PREOPERATIVE CONSIDERATIONS

The operating surgeon must use all the available resources of gathering information about the uterus and pelvis by thorough clinical examination and investigations to have a clear mind map of surgery. He should combine findings of pelvic examination with USG/MRI findings with exact mapping of location, size, no of fibroids, association of adenomyosis/endometriosis and scars of previous surgeries along with the lateral pelvic space. Operating surgeon must have very clear idea prior to VH for fibroid uterus of well thought of difficulties in advance and he should have plan ready to negotiate them. The standard technique of the surgeon may need to be modified depending upon these factors.

USG mapping comes handy to decide the surgical plan and MRI is rarely required. But MRI is more specific in deciding the nature of the uterine mass. Hence for any suspicious fibroid which has grown faster over last few months especially for a solitary, large fibroid it is necessary to differentiate it from sarcoma. Highly suspicious mass would influence the selection of the route of hysterectomy.

Many of these patients are anemic due to prolonged menorrhagia. Correction of preoperative anemia is necessary for increasing the surgical safety and for reducing post-operative morbidity. Intra venous iron therapy is very helpful in correcting anemia faster.

Consider preoperative GnRH analogues or SPRMs to shrink fibroids and reduce vascularity in selective cases. A few selective cases may benefit by this by converting them from being subjected to abdominal or laparoscopic route to vaginal route by reduction of the size of uterus. Also, a few months GnRH analogue therapy may help buy time for correction of anemia as these

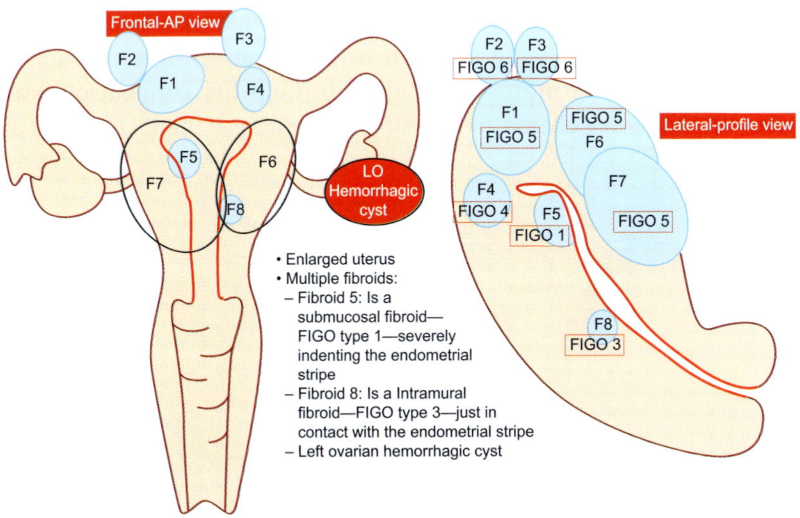

Fig. 2: Fibroid mapping on USG.
Courtesy: Dr Mayur Kulkarni

patients become amenorrheic on GnRH therapy. But it should not be used for all fibroid cases hoping to reduce size for surgical ease as results of this therapy are not consistent.

SURGICAL NUANCES

Exposure and Access

- Adequate vaginal access and good retraction are essential. Cases with narrow subpubic arch, morbid obesity and fixed, immobile uterus due to endometriosis pose serious problems.
- Weighted speculum, lateral retractors, and anterior wall retractor help visualization. A good surgical assistant with single bladed speculums of different width and lengths should suffice and should be readily available. These single blade speculums are versatile and can be used as lateral as well as anterior wall retractors.
- Hydro-dissection of anterior and posterior planes reduces tissue trauma although it may not be always necessary. In fact, authors never use it for their cases. We feel that it distorts the fascial anatomy. A few authors quote that it helps reduce the blood loss by controlling the oozing by tamponade effect. But if one dissects in a correct plane, inadvertent bleeding is not encountered.

Tips to Improve Access in the Earlier Part of the Surgery

The standard surgical steps for vaginal hysterectomy are followed which are described in detail in other chapter of this issue. Hence it is not described in detail here. Below are a few variations for cases with fibroid uteri.

Posterior colpotomy and accessing the cul-de-sac as a first step is advantageous in these cases. It allows for a thorough assessment of pelvis and the uterus by allowing surgeon to push one's finger through the colpotomy gathering more information to help his surgical planning. It gives the surgeon a chance to lyse flimsy adhesions if there are any. It also

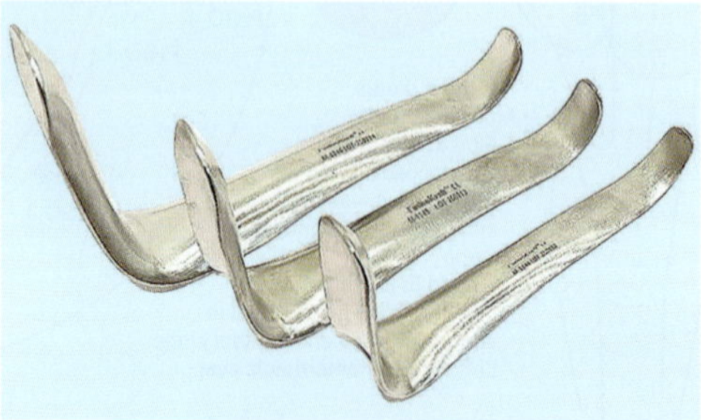

Fig. 3: Single bladed speculums.
Courtesy: Google image

allows for securing JUST uterosacral pedicles before proceeding with other surgical steps. By doing so one can achieve a descent of at least an inch. In case of NDVH, an inch of the descent the specimen can make further surgical journey easier by a mile.

Controlling Vascular Pedicles

One may not be able to access and open anterior peritoneum before ligating uterine vessels because of presence of fibroid/s on anterior wall. And it is not even necessary to do it at this stage of surgery. Ensuring that anterior vaginal wall is adequately mobilized and retracted antero-laterally while taking uterine vessel pedicles would help avoid bladder/ureteric injury. One needs to remember that lateral part of the bladder lies anterior to uterine vasculature and needs to be mobilized anterolaterally. One would be able to take uterine pedicles easily in most of the cases because uterine vessels always enter the uterus at the level of the isthmus. If one is able to secure utero-sacral ligaments he is already at the level of the isthmus. Once both the uterine artery pedicles are ligated or coagulated, blood loss will be minimized.

Another important tip is to take multiple small pedicles than to go for a big chunk of tissue even if it is lucrative to do so.

Bipolar energy or vessel sealing devices improve hemostasis. But be wary of the lateral spread of energy as no energy source is without lateral spread.

Uterine Mobilization

Fibroids come in all possible sizes, shapes and at all possible locations. Operating surgeon will face diverse and unique situations at every surgery asking for unique approach to each case. Hence one needs to be equipped with different approaches and skills to tackle these varied situations.

A pedunculated fibroid coming out of the cervix and projecting into the vagina needs to be removed at the beginning of the surgery. It may be small or as big as a fetal head. Twisting of the pedicle would serve the purpose in most of the cases without causing undue bleeding. A pedunculated fibroid arising from the lip of cervix can be clamped, ligated and cut before proceeding with the hysterectomy.

Cervical fibroid should not be a deterrent to attempt vaginal hysterectomy. It needs to be enucleated and removed before proceeding with clamping of pedicles. One can take a few stitches on the remaining fibroid capsule to restructure the cervix as it helps maintain anatomical orientation. If one is in the right plane, bleeding is minimal. One can use infiltration of diluted vasopressin here to achieve bloodless field.

For intramural, sub-mucous and sub-serosal fibroids one should proceed with standard technique as one would do for any other NDVH without bothering much about the size of the uterus. Just think about one pedicle at a time and one can successfully complete the surgery with patience and perseverance.

One needs to tackle the fibroid/s as they appear in the course of surgery using any of the previously thought of and practiced techniques like myomectomy, coring or morcellation of the fibroid. The choice of the technique depends upon the size of the fibroid. Smaller ones can be easily picked up and plucked out while larger ones (bigger than 6 cm) may need to be removed piecemeal using sharp knife or scalpel. A few surgeons prefer using myoma screw for myomectomy. One need not exert excessive dragging force on the myoma as it may help remove the myoma but sudden pressure changes in the pelvis may lead to avulsion or tearing of vascular pedicles leading to profuse bleeding.

Submucous fibroids are most easy to access. After securing uterine pedicles one can either transect the cervix or bisect the specimen till submucous fibroid is visible. Once visualized it can be removed by the different techniques mentioned above.

Sub-serosal fundal fibroids up to 8–10 cm size do not pose any difficult as one can easily secure the pedicles and complete hysterectomy and fibroid walks done along with the specimen. If the fundal fibroid is in close proximity to a cornu then it may make access to tubo-ovarian pedicle of that side difficult. In such situation one can complete the hysterectomy on the opposite side and pull the specimen in the vaginal cavity for ease of access to the side in question. One can also start morcellating the specimen from the side which is freed to debulk the specimen and to create space. Do remember that as you approach 'un-freed' cornu the bleeding from ovarian vessels starts and needs to be tackled in timely manner.

Larger sub-serosal fundal fibroids pose difficulty by the mere size restricting descent of the specimen into the vaginal canal. Disproportionately elongated cervix on pre-operative USG should raise a suspicion about this possibility where the specimen sits on the pelvic rim and denies to descend down in the vaginal canal.

Intramural fibroids are comparatively easy as they start "posing" as one proceeds with the hysterectomy as if asking to be removed. One can use well-rehearsed techniques of myomectomy, enucleation or morcellation of the fibroid as one starts to see them in the course of surgery.

Broad ligament fibroids are a special category. It is not a contraindication for vaginal approach. In fact, it is easier to access them vaginally than by any other route. Bony lateral pelvic walls prevent the spread of the fibroid laterally and push the fibroid medially towards vaginal canal. One can access the fibroid after clamping uterosacral and cardinal ligaments as one approaches the uterine vessel. Uterine vessel may lie below or above the fibroid. If it lies below, one can secure it before approaching the fibroid. If above, fibroid

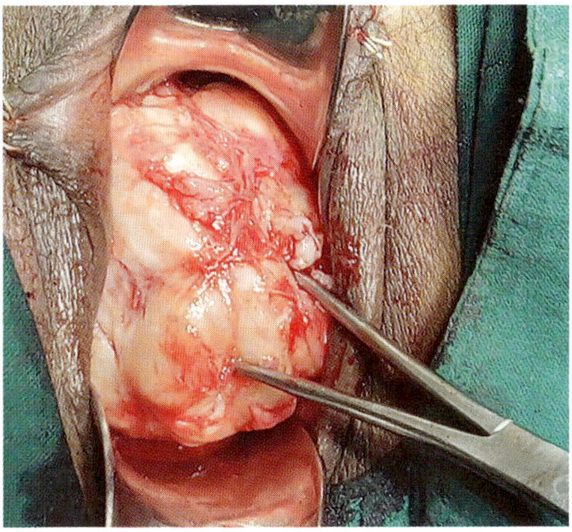

Fig. 4: Fibroid enucleation.
Courtesy: Dr Pankaj Sarode

needs to be removed first. In that case, avoid undue traction on the fibroid and be aware of the uterine vessel and the ureter which may be dragged with the fibroid . One needs to be aware of the ureter on opposite side also as a broad ligament fibroid on one side pushes the uterus on the opposite side reducing the distance between uterus and contralateral pelvic wall. Staying close to the specimen and being doubly sure before clamping is the key.

COMPLICATIONS: HOW TO AVOID THEM

Sharp dissection in the area of cervico-vesical fascia and not blunt pushing is the key to avoid bladder injury especially in case of previously scarred uterus. A fibroid at anterior lower segment may make access to the anterior peritoneal fold difficult. Go slow, try as much separation of the bladder from the lower segment as possible. Proceed with applying clamps bilaterally to achieve as much descent as possible and revisit the step of bladder separation. Repetition of these steps would help progress slowly and successfully. A bigger anterior wall fibroid may make access to the anterior peritoneum impossible. In that case one can achieve as much descent as possible by proceeding with the hysterectomy. One can secure uterine vessels in most of these cases. After securing uterine vessels one can start morcellating posterior uterine wall to access the fibroid posteriorly through the endometrial cavity. Once the fibroid is removed, anterior wall "falls down" creating a space between the anterior uterine wall and the pubic symphysis. At this stage one can proceed to opening of the anterior peritoneal fold in a standard fashion.

Ureteric injury during vaginal hysterectomy is rare but possible. Maintaining medial traction; staying as close to the uterine specimen as possible, avoiding excessive lateral energy spread and being aware of the ureter with high suspicion helps to avoid ureteric injury. Strict hemostasis to keep surgical field clean also helps to avoid ureteric injury by improved precision. One should avoid using energy for securing bleeding points on the lateral pelvic wall as ureters lie very close the point of action. It can be achieved by preemptive pedicle devascularization and meticulous stepwise technique. "Predictive anatomy" is a term coined by famous laparoscopic surgeon Dr Shailesh Puntambekar. We believe it is a surgical philosophy which helps prevent hemorrhagic complications and to achieve clean surgical field.

One needs to keep his surgical ego aside and treat each case as a trial VH keeping a plan ready to convert to another route when patient's safety is at stake.

CONCLUSION

Vaginal hysterectomy for uterine fibroids is safe and effective when supported by careful case selection and expertise. Mastery of surgical nuances allows VH to be performed even on moderately enlarged fibroid uteri.

Clinical judgement, skill, technique, experience and confidence of the surgeon are of utmost important to achieve success.

CHAPTER 5

Vagino-laparoscopic Hysterectomy for Very Large Fibroid Uteri: A Hybrid Strategy to Ease Surgical Challenges

Ramkrishna Purohit

INTRODUCTION

The vaginal route is the least invasive and most physiologic approach for hysterectomy, associated with shorter operative time, reduced hospital stay, and lower cost compared to laparoscopic or abdominal routes. However, the presence of a large fibroid uterus often makes the vaginal route technically difficult. While experienced surgeons can perform vaginal hysterectomy for uteri up to 16 weeks or more, there remains no clear upper limit. When the enlarged corpus resists descent or the adnexal pedicles are displaced, the risk of failed vaginal hysterectomy increases.

Total laparoscopic hysterectomy (TLH) and laparoscopic-assisted vaginal hysterectomy (LAVH) are accepted minimally invasive alternatives, yet both face distinct technical challenges in large uteri. A markedly enlarged uterus restricts exposure, displaces vascular pedicles, and complicates safe identification of anatomical planes. Thus, when both vaginal and laparoscopic approaches are expected to be difficult, combining their respective strengths can offer a safer hybrid option.

The concept of *vagino-laparoscopic hysterectomy (VLH)* involves initiating the procedure vaginally—completing devascularization up to the uterine arteries—followed by laparoscopic separation of upper pedicles and adnexa. This method reduces vascular load before laparoscopy, improves uterine mobility, and allows safe laparoscopic completion with minimal bleeding.

The present study aimed to evaluate the feasibility, safety, and outcomes of VLH for large fibroid uteri (≥16 weeks) in a prospective observational cohort at a private general hospital.

MATERIALS AND METHODS

Study Design and Participants

This observational study was conducted at *Purohit General Hospital, Odisha, India* between September 2020 and August 2022. Sixty-four consecutive patients undergoing hysterectomy for benign, non-prolapsed large fibroid uterus (≥16 weeks size) were included. Exclusion criteria were ventrofixed uterus and large cervical fibroids (>7.5 cm) with inaccessible cervix. Informed consent was obtained from all participants.

Study Parameters

Outcomes assessed included success rate of VLH, intraoperative technical challenges, blood loss, intraoperative and postoperative complications, and need for conversion. Descriptive statistics were used for analysis.

OPERATIVE TECHNIQUE

Vaginal Phase

The procedure began using the *Purohit technique* of vaginal hysterectomy. A 17 cm bipolar sealer–shearer was used to coagulate and divide structures. Sequentially, the vaginal wall, supravaginal and cardinal ligaments were separated from the cervix, and the posterior cul-de-sac was opened. The *uterosacral ligaments* were hooked and divided bilaterally, exposing the bulge of the *uterine artery*, which was then coagulated and divided between right-angle forceps.

The *uterovesical space* was dissected as far as possible. A Ryle's tube was introduced into the pelvis through the posterior cul-de-sac to allow pneumoperitoneum creation. Two roller gauze packs were placed to prevent gas leak, and a metal suction cannula was inserted into the uterine cavity for manipulation. The vaginal stump was clamped to reduce gas leak, and the surgeon proceeded to the laparoscopic phase.

Laparoscopic Phase

CO_2 insufflation was initiated through the Ryle's tube. Depending on uterine height, an umbilical or supraumbilical 10 mm primary port was introduced, followed by three 5 mm ports (bilateral lateral and suprapubic). Pneumoperitoneum was maintained at 10–12 mm Hg.

The vaginal assistant manipulated the uterine cannula upward and laterally, elevating the uterus and dislodging the lower segment from the narrow pelvis into the upper wider pelvis. This improved exposure and accessibility of displaced pedicles. Using bipolar sealer-shearer, the upper broad ligament, round ligaments, and cornual pedicles were coagulated and divided close to the uterine wall. The anterior and posterior leaf incisions were joined with the vaginally created dissections, completing the hysterectomy.

Opportunistic salpingectomy or *adnexectomy* was performed when indicated. The specimen was removed vaginally via morcellation, followed by laparoscopic lavage, and vaginal vault closure in two layers.

SPECIAL TECHNIQUES FOR CHALLENGING SITUATIONS

1. *Broad Ligament Elevation Technique:* For displaced uterine arteries not accessible vaginally, the lower broad ligament was elevated laterally with a suction cannula to expose and safely coagulate the artery close to the uterus, avoiding ureteric injury.

2. *Uterovesical Scar Elevation Technique:* In patients with thick uterovesical scarring from prior cesarean sections, the bladder wall was elevated to define the dissection plane, allowing stepwise separation under vision to prevent bladder injury.
3. *Laparoscopic Spiral Slimming:* In very large uteri, a spiral incision was made around the corpus using a bipolar shearer to reduce girth and ease vaginal extraction, without using a laparoscopic morcellator.

RESULTS

Sixty-four women underwent VLH for large fibroid uteri (≥16 weeks). The largest uterus corresponded to 26 weeks of gestation, with a mean specimen weight of *869.6 ± 275.1 g* (range 500–1900 g).

Intraoperative Observations

- *VLH success rate:* 63/64 cases (98.43%)
- *Conversion:* 1 case (1.56%) to mini-laparotomy for rectal adhesiolysis following prior myomectomy
- *No conversions* due to failed exposure or bleeding
- *No urinary tract or bowel injury.*

Vaginal separation of the uterosacral ligaments improved uterine mobility and laparoscopic ergonomics in all cases. Bilateral uterine arteries were successfully divided vaginally in *47 (73.43%)* patients. In *17 (26.56%)* cases where vaginal ligation was incomplete, the *broad ligament elevation technique* enabled successful laparoscopic division.

A thick uterovesical scar requiring the *scar elevation technique* was found in *7 (10.93%)* cases, all managed without bladder injury. Eight cases required laparoscopic spiral slimming for extraction.

Blood loss ranged from 300–900 mL in 25% cases; was less than 300 mL in other cases, no patient required conversion for uncontrolled bleeding. Postoperative recovery was uneventful in all patients.

DISCUSSION

Principal Findings

The VLH strategy combining vaginal devascularization and laparoscopic completion proved safe and effective for large uteri (≥16 weeks). The vaginal phase reduced uterine blood flow and increased mobility, simplifying laparoscopic ergonomics and visualization.

Traditional TLH or LAVH for large fibroid uteri often pose challenges due to restricted space, distorted anatomy, and displaced vascular pedicles. The VLH strategy effectively addressed these limitations. No case required conversion due to failed vascular exposure, contrasting with earlier studies reporting 5–10% conversion rates in large uteri (>1,000 g).

The *vaginal uterosacral detachment* elevated the uterus into the upper pelvis, creating a safer working field. The *broad ligament elevation* and *uterovesical scar elevation* techniques allowed secure dissection of displaced vessels and thick scars without retroperitoneal dissection or ureteric exposure. Consequently, no urinary tract injury occurred, even in cases with previous cesarean sections or large broad ligament fibroids.

CLINICAL IMPLICATIONS

VLH offers a reproducible, minimally invasive alternative for patients with large uteri where both pure vaginal and pure laparoscopic approaches are challenging. The hybrid route:

- Avoids excessive manipulation during TLH,
- Minimizes blood loss by early uterine artery control,
- Prevents ureteric injury by keeping dissection close to the uterus,
- Facilitates safe removal of large specimens vaginally, and
- Eliminates the need for power morcellation.

Furthermore, it can be performed in low-resource settings using standard laparoscopic instruments and a bipolar shearer.

TECHNICAL CONSIDERATIONS

The use of *bipolar sealer-shearer* both vaginally and laparoscopically provided precise hemostasis without sutures, enabling efficient devascularization. Surgeons trained in vaginal hysterectomy can adapt easily to this approach with moderate laparoscopic skill.

LIMITATIONS

This was a single-center observational study without a control group. The learning curve for the vaginal bipolar shearer technique must be considered. Comparative studies with TLH or LAVH for large uteri could further validate its advantages.

KEY MASSAGE

- The *vagino-laparoscopic hysterectomy (VLH)* is a safe, effective, and minimally invasive hybrid strategy for large fibroid uteri (≥16 weeks). By initiating surgery vaginally to devascularize the uterus and complete upper pedicle separation laparoscopically, this approach significantly eases technical challenges, enhances exposure, minimizes blood loss, and reduces the risk of urinary tract injury.
- VLH can be adopted in most large uteri where traditional routes pose difficulty, combining the ergonomic benefits of laparoscopy with the natural access advantages of the vaginal route.

SUGGESTED READING

1. Aarts JW, Nieboer TE, Johnson N, Tavender E, Garry R, Mol BW, et al. Surgical approach to hysterectomy for benign gynaecological disease. Cochrane Database Syst Rev. 2015;2015(8):CD003677.
2. Cianci S, Gueli Alletti S, Rumolo V, Rosati A, Rossitto C, Cosentino F, et al. Total laparoscopic hysterectomy for enlarged uteri: factors associated with the rate of conversion to open surgery. J Obstet Gynaecol. 2019;39:805-10.
3. Fashokun TB, Honda VL. Vaginal hysterectomy. In: Handa VL, Linda VL (Eds). Telinde's Operative Gynaecology, 12th edition. Philadelphia: Wolters Kluwer; 2015. pp. 358-9.
4. Kho RM, Abrão MS. In search for the best minimally invasive hysterectomy approach for the large uterus: a review. Clin Obstet Gynecol. 2017;60:286-95.
5. Purohit RK. Purohit technique of vaginal hysterectomy: a new approach. BJOG. 2003;110(12):1115-9.
6. Sandberg EM, Twijnstra ARH, Driessen SRC, Jansen FW. Total Laparoscopic Hysterectomy Versus Vaginal Hysterectomy: A Systematic Review and Meta-Analysis. J Minim Invasive Gynecol. 2017;24(2):206-17.
7. Uccella S, Kho RM, Garzon S, Casarin J, Zorzato PC, Ghezzi F. The Large Uterus Classification System: a prospective observational study. BJOG. 2021;128:1526-33.

6 CHAPTER

Le Forte's Colpocleisis

RM Saraogi, Sonam Kataria

INTRODUCTION

In a medical context "colpo", is a prefix derived from the Greek word for "kolpos" meaning hollow, fold or womb, and it refers to the vagina. "Cleisis" is a medical term meaning surgical closure or obliteration of an opening, often used as a suffix in medical words. For example, colpocleisis is a surgical procedure to close the vaginal canal.

TYPES OF OBLITERATIVE SURGERIES

- Partial colpocleisis
- Total colpocleisis
- Introital tightening

PRINCIPLES OF SURGERY

- To close the vagina partially or completely with the prolapse reduced above.
- These surgeries are generally carried out in a very old post-menopausal high-risk patients where anesthesia is contraindicated.
- It should be done in patients who does not desire sexual function.
- There should not be any uterine or pelvic pathology.

INDICATIONS

- Old postmenopausal women patient with 3rd degree uterine prolapse with unhealthy cervix
- Sexual function is not desired
- Medically unfit for surgery
- Vault prolapses

CONTRAINDICATIONS

- Patient with intact uterus who is not menopause
- Bad cervix, uterine pathology
- Patient desires sexual intercourse

We cannot have a cafeteria approach in prolapse surgeries.
The operative technique should be combined with appropriate clinical examination to obtain maximum benefit to the patients.

LE FORTE'S COLPOCLEISIS PROCEDURE

- Denudation of rectangular vaginal flaps from anterior and posterior vaginal walls.
- Apposition of the denuded anterior and posterior vaginal walls, the reduction progresses step by step with placing of the sutures and when two surfaces are united throughout the reduction of complete walls.
- Ancillary surgery which can be performed with this is perineorrhaphy which gives good support to perineum.
- SUI surgery in the form of Kelly stitch, meshplasty, TVT, and TOT can be performed.

ADVANTAGES

- Can be performed under local anesthesia or Xylocard
- It is very simple
- Can be performed rapidly
- Gives good satisfactory results
- Can be performed with 3rd degree uterine descent with cystocele, rectocele
- Can be performed in cases of procidentia
- Can be performed in vaginal vault prolapse. Repair.
- Success rate for Le Forte's is above 95% and post operative pain is minimal.

DISADVANTAGES

- It can result in SUI
- Hematoma formation can occur.

IN NUTSHELL

A: After menopause

B: Blood loss negligible

C: Comorbidity diabetes, heart diseases, hypertension, unfit for anesthesia

D: Damage to adjacent organs is negligible

E: Economic

F: Fast recovery no failure

G: Good

H: Hospitalization 1–2 days

I: Instruments–nil

J: Juna technique but forgotten

K: Knowledge – first poster can do it

L: Low morbidity local anesthesia

M: Mortality nil, menopause

N: No pain

O: Obese patient old age

P: Postmenopausal, painless

Q: Quick recovery

R: Recurrence nil

S: No scar sexual function not possible

Sui yes can occur, simple underutilized

T: Time can be done in less time

U: Understanding is easy

V: Very effective

W: Working gives more satisfactory, wound infection less.

SUGGESTED READING

1. Buchsbaum GM, Lee TG. Vaginal Obliterative Procedures for Pelvic Organ Prolapse: A Systematic Review. Obstet Gynecol Surv. 2017;72(3):175-83.
2. Felder L, Heinzelmann-Schwarz V, Kavvadias T. How does colpocleisis for pelvic organ prolapse in older women affect quality of life, body image, and sexuality? A critical review of the literature. Womens Health (Lond). 2022;18:17455057221111067.
3. Raju R, Kisby CK, Occhino JA. Teaching the art of LeFort colpocleisis: a moderate-fidelity, low-cost simulation model. Int Urogynecol J. 2021;32(8):2295-9.
4. Welch EK, Dengler KL, Wheat JE, Heuer CW, Trikhacheva AS, Gruber DD, et al. Colpocleisis Techniques: An Open-and-shut Case for Advanced Pelvic Organ Prolapse. Urology. 2023;176:252.

7 CHAPTER

High Utero Sacral Ligament Suspension: A Novel Native Tissue Support for POP

Uma Rani Swain, Sandhya Panigrahi

INTRODUCTION

Majority of pelvic organ prolapse begin with apical descent which carry uterus and cervix down and gradually descend further taking lower 2/3rd of vagina. So the success of surgical procedure primarily depends on effective apical support in addition to repair of other compartments. There are number of surgical options to address the apical prolapse.

Routes are both Vaginal and abdominal:

- *Vaginal methods:* Native tissue repair/with mesh
- *Abdominal (laparotomy/laparoscopy/robotic):* Sling/mesh can be used as prosthesis

ETIOLOGY/GENESIS OF POP

Uterus has number of ligaments and fasciae for its support, which surrounds the cervix at the level of internal os known as *peri-cervical ring*. It holds and stabilizes the uterus in pelvis at the level of ischial spine and create all four fornices in relation with vagina.

With the process of aging, child births and estrogen deficiency during menopause, the pelvic floor structures including muscles and endo pelvic fascia loses its tone and strength. It fails to provide a strong platform to keep pelvic organs in place. In addition pelvic ligaments also get attenuated, stretched and weak allowing the pelvic organs to descend gradually into the vagina and then outside introitus given rise to different stages of prolapse depend on the levels of vaginal support.

Conservative managements in form of nutritional supplements, pelvic floor muscle rehabilitation and vaginal pessary are considerably effective in early stages but not proved effective in treating higher stages of POP. Surgical correction remains the main modality of treatment in such cases.

PRINCIPLE OF APICAL SUPPORT

When the uterine supports become defective, other pelvic ligaments are taken into help for reconstruction procedure. These ligaments are being selected according their strength and position in relation to the prolapse organs, which acts like new support.

In direct suspension procedures, the selected ligament should be close to the vault. Whereas in indirect (mesh) surgery it is the distant ligament which supports the prolapse through a piece of mesh.

PRINCIPLE OF HIGH UTEROSACRAL LIGAMENT SUSPENSION (HUSLS)

It is a direct type of support, in which the intermediate (middle) portion of USL is selected for suspension. In case of uterine descent the distal part of USL attached to cervix and vagina gets stretched and attenuated and becomes ineffective to support, whereas the mid part remain unchanged in its structure both in length and strength and therefore, suitable for an effective support.

Mainly two subtypes of USL suspension are advocated:

1. *Point suspension* in which series of permanent sutures are passed through the substance of the mid part of USL, which then is taken out of ipsilateral angle of vault. When finally tied the vaginal apex gets lifted up, and remains fixed permanently.
2. *Plication* of USL by continuous running suture through intermediate and distal part of ligament which ends with the angle of vault. When suture get tied the, the lower 2/3rd of USL gets compressed with lifting up the vault high inside the pelvic cavity.

Both types of procedure are bilateral in nature as a result of which the length, caliber and the anatomical axis of vaginal canal are well maintained.

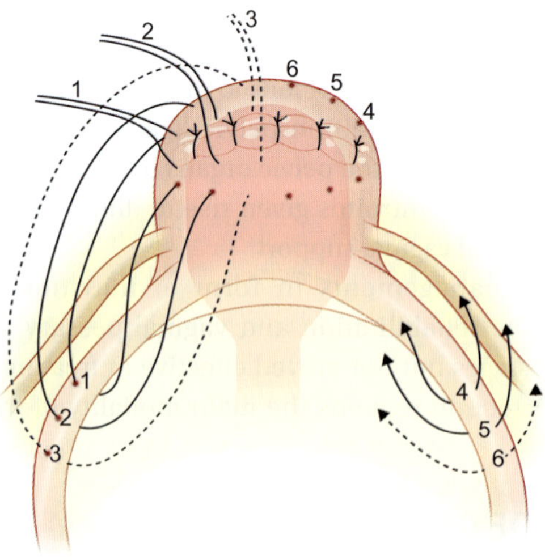

Fig. 1: The series of suture passage through USL and taken out of vault.

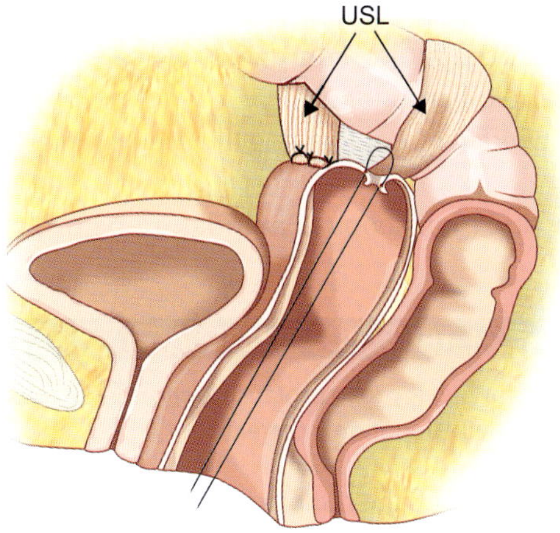

Fig. 2: Normal axis of vagina following procedure.

ADVANTAGES OF HIGH USL SUSPENSION

- Use of patient's own native tissue is always better than artificial synthetic prosthesis like mesh and sling.
- As USL has good length so the point of suspension can be manipulated according to the available vaginal length.
- Anatomical axis of vagina and natural suppleness are maintained which also favor sexual function in addition.
- Complications like mesh erosion, extrusion, infection and tissue avulsion are not there in this procedure.
- It is a highly effective and durable method and its effects can be comparable to abdominal mesh colpopexy.

COMPARISON WITH SSLS AND MESH COLPOPEXY

- Mainly defer in maintaining the vaginal axis. In SSLS because of its unilateral nature the 9 gets deviated to one side and also placed deep down in pelvis.
- SSLS is equally effective procedure comparable with HUSLS
- Both of these native tissue suspension require the presence of good vaginal length to keep the vault in high position.
- Unlike native tissue, abdominal mesh can be used even in short vagina and also mesh itself has better strength than native tissue ligament.
- Drawback of mesh or sling is its nature of healing by fibrosis which can make the vagina a rigid structure, may not be suitable for sexual function.

COMPLICATION

- *USL* doesn't carry any major blood vessels or nerve so hemorrhage or nerve related complication are rare.

- As ureter runs parallel to USL in its lower 2/3rd of its course, the said procedure carries the major complications with ureter in the form of kinking, injury and obstruction.
- It can be easily avoided by conforming the ureteric patency through check cystoscopy.
- Intra-op diagnostic cystoscopy is mandatory before completion of the procedure.

TAKE-HOME MESSAGE

- High USL suspension for pelvic organ prolapse is considered to be a highly effective and durable procedure which not only corrects the prolapse, but also allows sexual function.
- Being a native tissue, it avoids the complication related to mesh.
- The only complication lies with ureters, which can be mastered with anatomical knowledge and surgical skills.

SUGGESTED READING

1. Alfahmy A, Mahran A, Conroy B, Brewka RR, Ibrahim M, Sheyn D, et al. Abdominal and vaginal pelvic support with concomitant hysterectomy for uterovaginal pelvic prolapse: a comparative systematic review and meta-analysis. Int Urogynecol J. 2021;32(8):2021-31.
2. Campagna G, Vacca L, Panico G, Vizzielli G, Caramazza D, Zaccoletti R, et al. Laparoscopic High Uterosacral Ligament Suspension vs. Laparoscopic Sacral Colpopexy for Pelvic Organ Prolapse: A Case-Control Study. Front Med (Lausanne). 2022;9:853694.
3. Chen Y, Peng L, Zhang J, Shen H, Luo D. Sacrospinous Ligament Fixation vs Uterosacral Ligaments Suspension for Pelvic Organ Prolapse: A Systematic Review and Meta-Analysis. Urology. 2022;166:133-9.
4. Novara L, Sgro LG, Pecchio S, Ottino L, Tomatis V, Biglia N. Transvaginal high uterosacral ligament suspension: An alternative to McCall culdoplasty in the treatment of pelvic organ prolapse. Eur J Obstet Gynecol Reprod Biol. 2019;240:278-81.

8 CHAPTER

Obstetric Perineal Trauma and Oasis

Mohan A Gadam, Nikita Gadam

INTRODUCTION

We see OASI and perineal trauma as a commonest surgical intervention on females and bring to us a major health issue especially in country like ours where the confinements are in big numbers. Almost all (85–90%) of women delivering in India suffer from perineal trauma and many land up with OASIS (5–10%). Literature review gives the incidence as 5.7 % of all primigravids.

Given the number of deliveries occurring all over the world, this is undoubtedly a major health hazard. It takes a big toll on the health professionals and a financial burden on the authorities.

Most women who suffer from OASIS remain silent as it's a big social stigma, and often do not seek medical advice due to cost constrains and immense tolerance. Few remain asymptomatic. However, all of these women are at risk of developing complications with advancing age and with future confinements.

All these affected women should be identified and be given special care so that they do not suffer in future.

These women should have access to all traditional methods of managements. They should also be offered certain advance diagnostic technologies if available.

Any anal sphincter injury occurring at the time of delivery should certainly be diagnosed immediately and also be treated immediately. It would be a gold standard to perform per rectal examination after each and every delivery to rule out OASIS. The famous writing in one of the postgraduate book is: If you don't put your finger in it then you are putting your foot in to it. As once diagnosed, primary repair is the main stay of surgical intervention.

Fecal incontinence resulting from an undiagnosed OASI can be addressed by both conservative and operative measures.

ESTABLISHED RISK FACTORS FOR OASIS (NIH 2021)

- Operative vaginal deliveries (Forceps, vacuum, IPVs)
- Midline episiotomies
- All primigravidas

- High infant birth weight (>4 kg)
- Prolonged second stage of labor
- Advanced maternal age
- Asian ethnicity
- Persistent occiput posterior position
- Induction of labor
- Epidural analgesia
- Shoulder dystocia
- These risk factors are mostly inherent to the process itself and hence can't be altered.
- There are some preventive measures which can be adopted by all of us. But they do not yield substantial benefit. Few of them are listed below:
  - Some protective obstetric maneuvers.
  - Continuous perineal message and protection
  - Warm compression on the perineum in the second stage of labor appear to reduce the risk of OASIS.
  - Vaginal deliveries, however, are the most common cause of perineal trauma.
  - It was always thought that episiotomy would prevent these complications. Hence there was a concept of universal episiotomy for many decades. This is now not an accepted principle. Restricted use of episiotomy is the norm all over the world.
  - It's a gold standard for all of us to make restricted use episiotomies and that to medio-lateral with 45–60 degrees angle from the Fourchette (midline), only when it is required.

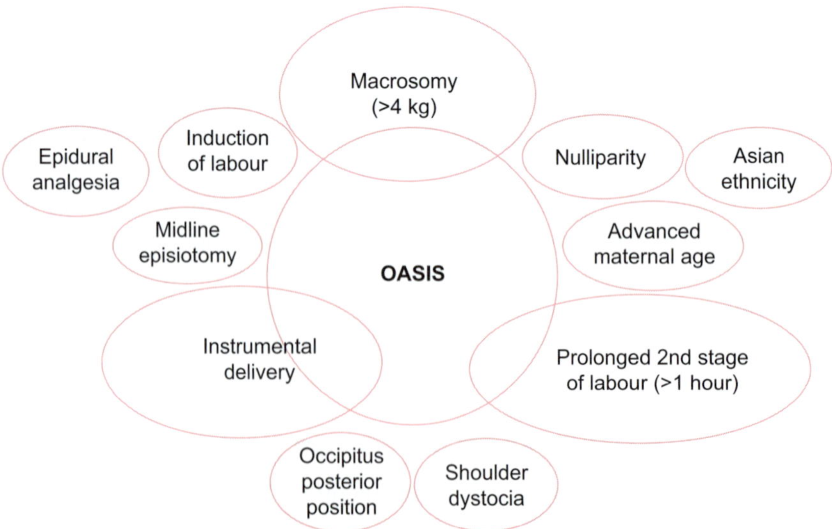

Fig. 1: Diagrammatic presentation of risk factors for OASIS.

OASIS and perineal trauma is known following many other conditions. Pelvic injuries and fractures, sexual assaults and forceful sexual intercourse, and other iatrogenic injuries, that can potentially lead to sphincter damage.

Anterior perineal traumas (labia majora and minora, anterior vagina, urethra, or clitoris), are not associated with lethal injuries and are easily manageable with conventional modes of treatment. However it is posterior trauma which is more morbid immediately as well as on long term basis and are difficult to manage.

Perineal trauma cause following defects and deficiencies:

- Anatomical defects and disruptions which may include OASIS.
- Neurogenic damage of pelvic nerves with it is long term sequels.
- Pudendal nerve is often the victim of overstretching and the compression of the neuro-vascular bundle finally leading to denervation.
- Diagnosis of these injuries is challenging and complex often leading to no results.

There are a few newer modalities for diagnosing above defects with limited sensitivity. Some are used in modern day managements but many arc not worth considering:

1. Endo-anal ultrasound (EAUS)
2. MRI
3. EMG
4. Transperineal ultrasound (TPUS)

None of the above modalities are of great value in optimizing the outcome or diagnosing the conditions. There future ability to improve the outcome is also questionable. Besides most of the neurological injuries resolve spontaneously.

OASIS

Now a day there is lot of debate on this topic. Much attention is given to prevent these injuries, given the number of deliveries all over the world. However, there is an inherent risk involved in the process of delivery itself. OASIS accounts to about 0.5 and 17%. The risk is much more in primiparous patients than in multiparous patients.

Long-term risk associated with vaginal delivery are:

- Urinary incontinence,
- Fecal incontinence
- Pelvic organ prolapse.

Above diagnostic tests are sparingly used, most of us have no access to them and their sensitivity is really questionable. These methods are not evolved as yet. It is in fact debatable as to how much importance to be given to them.

TABLE 1: Diagnosis of obstetric anal sphincter injuries (new evidence and prospective).

Diagnostic test	*Target*	*Sensitivity*	*Accuracy*	*Reproducibility*	*Non-Op. dependence*	*Intra-operative use*
Traditional						
EAUS	Morphology	++	++	–	–	+
Anorectal manometry	Function	+	+	+	+	–
MRI	Morphology	++	++	++	++	–
Experimental						
TPUS	Morphology	+	+	–	–	+
Impedance spectroscopy	Morphology function	+	+	++	++	

EAUS

- EAUS (Endo-anal ultra-sonography) is the most studied and used in the diagnosis and management of OASIS. It can detect both external and internal anal sphincter injuries. It is used at many higher centers including India
- Three-dimensional EAUS (3D-EAUS) can even detect smaller defects which may not be detected by EAUS. High end machines are available all over in India.
- Diagnostic ability of EAUS being very high, with high sensitivity and predictive value has considerable prognostic value and is most commonly used methodology.
- This modality is reasonably safe and can assess the perineum and OASIS and is often well accepted by most of the patients.
- EAUS has a good prognostic value and is also a useful tool intra operatively. As it can pin point the exact site of defect and hence can assist in surgical settings.
- EAUS can also give sufficient idea about long term prognosis and hence can be used during follow-up period.
- It can also give idea about patients at high risk of developing long term complications.
- However with all possible knowledge, role of EAUS is not yet clearly defined in the management of OASIS.
- EAUS may also be helpful in diagnosing patients at risk of developing future complications, there by planning the mode of delivery in a given patient.

TPUS

- Trans perineal ultra-sonography (TPUS) is still in developmental stage and its applications are not so far well-defined. It primarily involves use of high-frequency curved array transducer on the perineum (trans-perineal or trans-labial), for assessment the anatomy of the pelvic floor and to also diagnose anal sphincter dynamics and pathologies.
- Below are the TPUS images of normal anal sphincter complex and those of a damaged one.

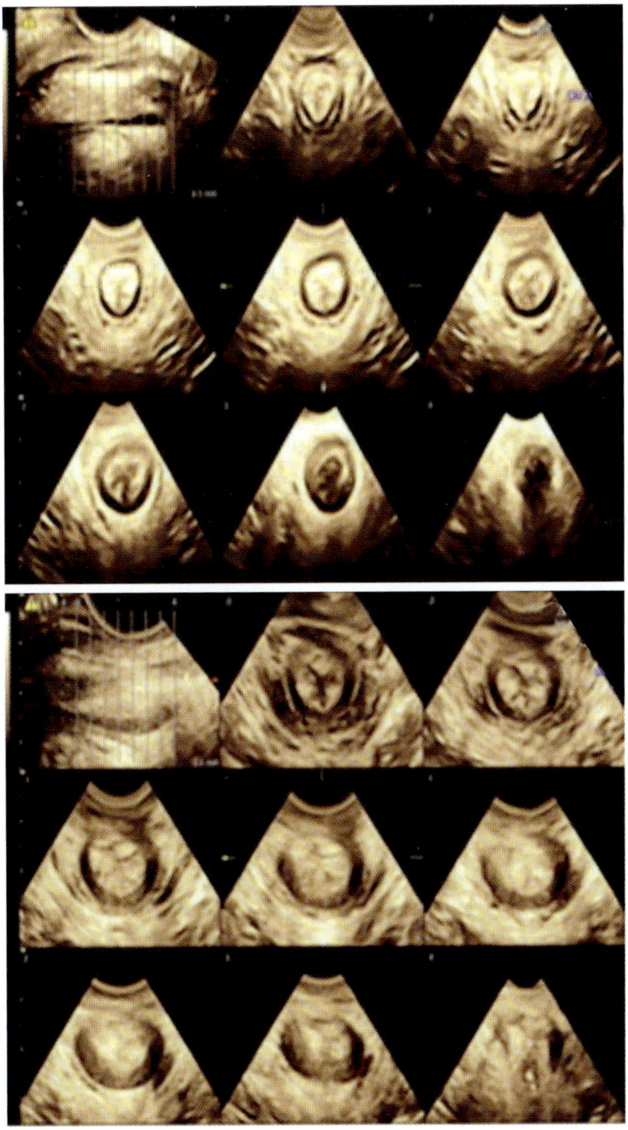

Fig. 2: TPUS Images.

TIAS AND TEAS (TPUS)

- Tomographic ultrasound imaging of internal (IAS) and external anal sphincter (EAS) as shown in the diagram above can detect the tears in external and internal sphincters. Exact site and the degree of defect can be assessed.
- The EAS appears as a ring of hyper echogenicity surrounding the thin hypoechogenic ring of the IAS.
- The mucosal folds of the anal canal is in the center of the image as shown.
- Sphincters are normal in all the transverse slices of the left picture (complete rings).
- The picture on the right show a full-thickness defect of both sphincters (both concentric rings are interrupted).
- If one compares EAUS to TPUS, later has the advantages of being more accessible, relatively less invasive, and it is more acceptable by the patient, it involves no insertion of the transducer in anal canal (exo-anal).
- TPUS is thus becoming more and more popular in recent years. However, this modality does not give panoramic view of the images and does not differentiate tissues as well as in EAUS. Hence this modality is not well accepted so far.
- More and more studies are thus required to prove the superiority of TPUS over TAUS. Further research is required in this regard. But a time will come where TPUS will be a better modality over TAUS as it is less invasive.
- TAUS and TPUS are still not accepted as diagnostic tools for OASIS.
- Inter-observer variations, lack of expertise and doubtful accuracy limits the use of these modalities in management of OASI.

MRI

- MRI is fairly useful in diagnosing EAS injuries. But not so good in diagnosing IAS.
- External phased array MRI can diagnose both EAS as well as IAS injuries.
- MRI has the advantages of being non-invasive, reproducible, not operator-dependent.
- In centers where EAUS is not available while MRI is, it may help in making the diagnosis, particularly if there is concern for a fistula.
- Dynamic MR defecography is another option for study of pelvic floor disorders, advantage being it is non-invasive and the availability of MRI all over.
- In nutshell for anatomic defects EAUS and MRI suits, and for functional defects anorectal manometry is better.
- Dynamic MRI defecography is better used for patients complaining of fecal incontinence which is a part of end-stage descending perineal syndrome. It would then change the surgical approach.

Flowchart 1: Perineal trauma.

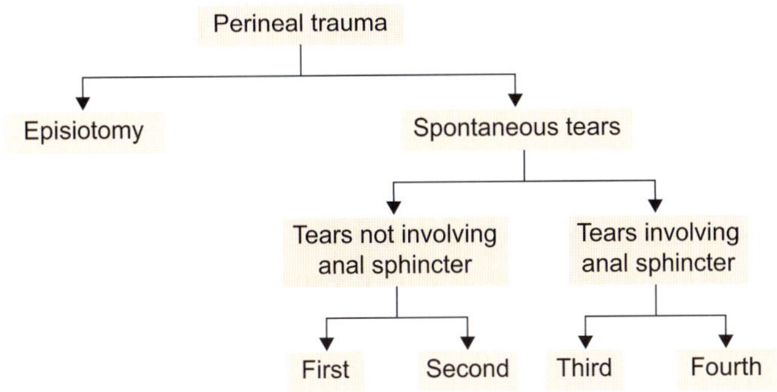

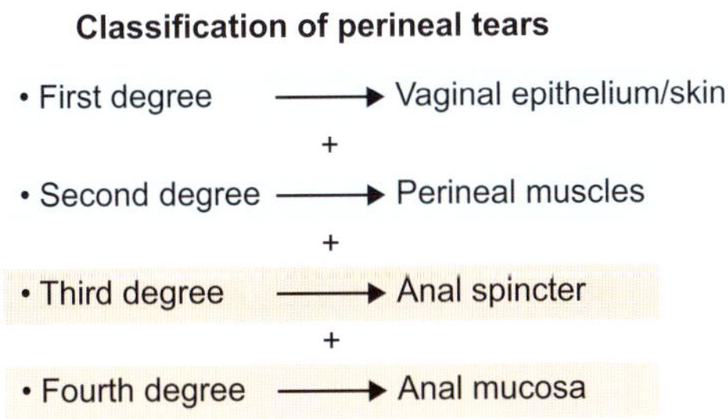

Fig. 3: Perineal tears related to deliveries/spontaneous or operative.

CLASSIFICATION OF 3RD AND 4TH DEGREE PERINEAL INJURY (RCOG GUIDELINES)

3rd degree: Anal sphincter tears

3a: <50% external sphincter thickness

3b: >50% external sphincter thickness

3c: Internal sphincter torn

4th degree: Anal epithelium torn.

Why to Repair Perineal Trauma?

- To control bleeding
- To prevent infection
- To prevent anal incontinence in 3rd and 4th degree

Nonsuturing of 1st and 2nd Degree Tears: Evidence

- 1st and 2nd degree un-sutured associated with poorer wound healing, and associated fibrosis
- Increases risk of dyspareunia.
- Defeats cosmetic scar

Prerequisites for Suturing Perineal Tear

- Thorough vaginal and rectal examination to check extent of perineal trauma, involvement of perineal muscles, anal sphincter and finally involvement of anal or rectal wall.
- Check instruments, suture pack, materials.
- Local infiltration is done with 1% lignocaine.
- Injections through the skin are best avoided.
- Always call for help as the assistance of experienced Obstetrician is always best.

Suturing Technique

Standard age old technique is the closure in three layers. First layer is the vaginal mucosa. Suturing is done with continuous non interlocking stitch, the first stitch is going well beyond the apex and continuing till perineal skin. Do not tighten the stitch too much which will otherwise give rise to sever pain and the wound will heal with fibrosis.

Second layer are series of interrupted sutures so as to get the muscles of perineal pouch and the subcutaneous tissue in opposition and to have a perfect anatomical closure.

Final layer is the suturing of perineal skin with interrupted mattress stitches. The best suture material is delayed absorbable suture like Vicryl rapid. Good old days this suturing was done with Chromic catgut, which is used even now at many centers in India. I am not a strong proponent of Chronic catgut, as it gets absorbed fast, it has less tensile strength and in presence of infection it easily undergoes proteolytic digestion. Only advantage is that it being cheaper and cost cutting. This is a rat race and every few years better and better suture materials will be available and the companies will promote their products. We should hence take an appropriate decision looking at the circumstances.

What is Advocated by Latest Guidelines and Level 1 Evidence?

Suturing of vaginal mucosa:

- Identify the apex of the vaginal wound
- Close the vaginal skin with a loose continuous stitch
- At the fourchette insert the needle through the skin to emerge in the center of the perineal trauma.

Suturing muscle layer:

- Check the depth of the trauma—it may be necessary to insert two layers of sutures
- Close the perineal muscle with a continuous non-locking stitch—taking care not to leave any dead space

Suturing of perineal skin:

- At the inferior end of the wound bring the needle out under the skin surface
- Stitches placed below the skin surface in the SC layer—thus avoiding the profusion of nerve endings
- Take bites of tissue from each side of the wound until the hymenal remnants are reached
- Secure the finished repair with a loop knot tied in the vagina.

Please kindly note that there is *Level 1a evidence for use of* Vicryl rapide suture material & The continuous non-locking technique for perineal repair- all layers.

Why continuous technique?

- No knots, Sutures accommodate themselves to swelling as it occurs
- Tight sutures cause pain especially if the wound becomes edematous—may cause tissue hypoxia and delay healing
- Skin sutures inserted into subcutaneous layer thus avoiding nerve endings in skin surface—less pain
- Economical—single suture used.

CLASSIFICATION OF 3RD AND 4TH DEGREE PERINEAL TEARS: OASIS (OBSTETRIC ANAL SPHINCTER INJURIES)

RCOG Guidelines

3rd degree: Anal sphincter tear

3a: <50% external sphincter thickness

3b: > 50% external sphincter thickness

3c: Internal sphincter torn

4th degree: Anal epithelium torn

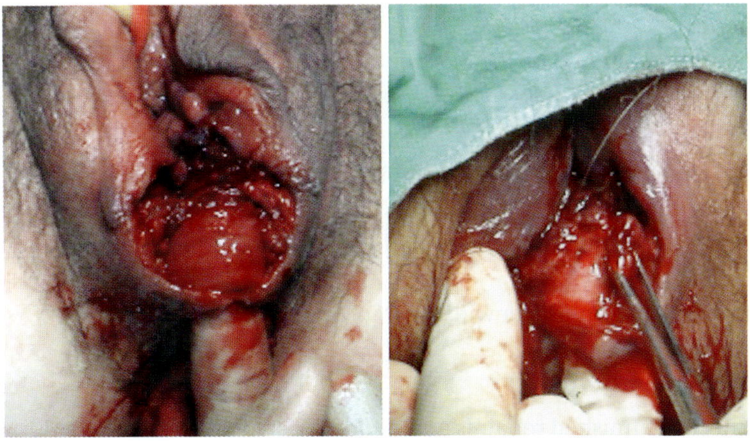

Fig. 4: Anal sphincters.

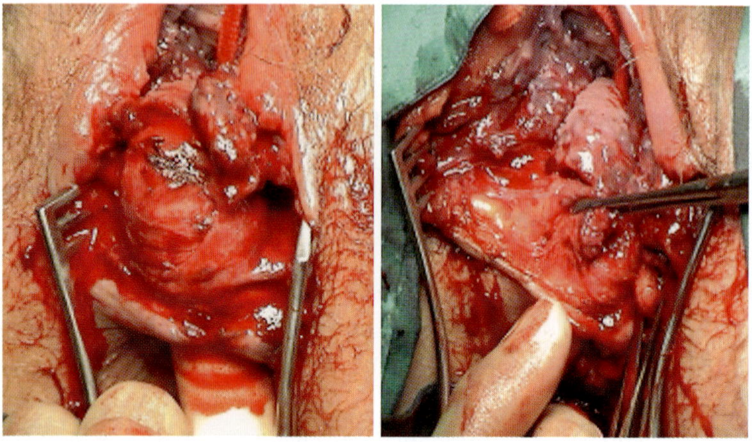

Fig. 5: Sphincter identification.

SUTURING OF 3RD AND 4TH DEGREE PERINEAL TEARS

One must adhere to basic principles of surgery, all through the procedure. A senior Obstetrician well worst with the procedure should always be called for a repair or for help. Procedure should be performed in a major operation theatre.

- Thorough clinical evaluation, EUA, should be performed.
- The extent of damage be evaluated properly.
- Per rectal examination is the key to identify the defect and extent of damage.
- Parts are painted and draped.
- Self-retaining catheter in inserted.
- Meticulous hemostasis, thorough asepsis and anatomical closure are the hallmarks of this repair.
- Always do a per rectal examination at the end to ensure that the repair is perfect
- First repair should be the best repair.

Suturing Technique

- Anal mucosa is best sutured with interrupted vicryl 3-0 with knots in anal canal.
- Internal anal sphincter is sutured with mattress end to end sutures with 3-0 PDS or 2-0 vicryl.
- External anal sphincter with 3-0 PDS or 2-0 vicryl suture

Immediate Postop

- Check the finished repair is anatomically correct.
- Complete hemostasis is achieved.

- Two finger vaginal examination is easily possible.
- PR examination is must to confirm the intact repair.
- Check swabs and instruments
- Proper documentation and notes to detail out entire procedure.
- Pain relief
- Discuss diet, hygiene pelvic floor exercises.

Postoperative Management

- Adequate Appropriate Broad spectrum antibiotics (cefuroxime 1500 mg. and metronidazole 500 mg) – To be administered IV intra operatively.
- And continued orally for a week.
- Stool softeners.
- Soft or full diet from day one.
- Pelvic floor exercises for 6 to 12 weeks following repair
- Review after 6 to 12 weeks
- Symptomatic patients should be subjected EAUS and anorectal manometry.
- Advisable to follow-up for at least 12 months

Recommended Practice

- Rectal examination after every delivery.
- Classify the perineal injuries accurately
- Analgesia/anesthesia as appropriate
- *Evidence based practice:* Use of appropriate materials and methods
- *Trained person to undertake the repair:* Recognition of own limitations
- Training programs and supervision of perineal repairs for all levels.

This article does not cover management of old healed perineal tear repairs. Also it does not cover other procedures like use of bulbospongiosus grafts and gracilis muscle grafts.

We will end here by quoting the famous words from TeLende's text book: If you don't put your finger in it, you will then have to put your foot in to it.

SUGGESTED READING

1. Aasheim V, Nilsen ABV, Reinar LM, Lukasse M. Perineal techniques during the second stage of labour for reducing perineal trauma. Cochrane Database Syst Rev. 2017;6:CD006672.
2. Abdool Z, Sultan AH, Thakar R. Ultrasound imaging of the anal sphincter complex: A review. Br J Radiol. 2012;85:865-75.
3. Adams EJ, Bricker L, Richmond DH, Neilson JP. Systematic review of third degree tears: Risk factors. Int Urogynecol J Pelvic Floor Dysfunct. 2001;12 (Suppl. 3):12.
4. Alavi K, Chan S, Wise PH, Kaiser AM, Sudan R, Bordeianou L. Fecal Incontinence: Etiology, Diagnosis, and Management. J Gastrointest Surg. 2015;19:1910-21.

5. Albuquerque A. Endoanal ultrasonography in fecal incontinence: Current and future perspectives. World J Gastrointest Endosc. 2015;7:575-81.
6. Allen R, Hosker GL, Smith ARB, Warrell DW. Pelvic floor damage and childbirth: A neurophysiological study. BJOG Int J Obstet Gynaecol. 1990;97:770-9.
7. Andrews V, Sultan AH, Thakar R, Jones PW. Occult anal sphincter injuries—Myth or reality? BJOG Int J Obstet Gynaecol. 2006;113:195-200.
8. Andrews V, Thakar R, Sultan AH. Structured hands on training in repair of obstetric anal sphincter injuries: An audit of clinical practice. Int Urogynecol J Pelvic Floor Dysfunct. 2009;20:193-9.
9. Baghestan E, Irgens LM, Børdahl PE, Rasmussen S. Trends in Risk Factors for Obstetric Anal Sphincter Injuries in Norway. Obstet Gynecol. 2010;116:25-34.
10. Barbosa M, Christensen P, Møller-Bek K, Brogaard L, Glavind-Kristensen M. Can ultrasound 10 days after obstetric anal sphincter injury predict anal incontinence at long-term follow-up? Int Urogynecol J. 2021:1-10.
11. Borycka-Kiciak K, Młyńczak M, Kiciak A, Pietrzak P, Dziki A. Non-invasive obstetric anal sphincter injury diagnostics using impedance spectroscopy. Sci Rep. 2019;9:7097.
12. Carrington EV, Heinrich H, Knowles CH, Fox M, Rao S, Altomare DF, et al. The international anorectal physiology working group (IAPWG) recommendations: Standardized testing protocol and the London classification for disorders of anorectal function. Neurogastroenterol Motil. 2020;32:e13679.
13. Carroli G, Mignini L. Episiotomy for vaginal birth. Cochrane Database Syst Rev. 2009:CD000081.
14. Cattani L, Neefs L, Verbakel JY, Bosteels J, Deprest J. Obstetric risk factors for anorectal dysfunction after delivery: A systematic review and meta-analysis. Int Urogynecol J. 2021:1–12.
15. Coats PM, Chan KK, Wilkins M, Beard RJ. A comparison between midline and mediolateral episiotomies. BJOG Int J Obstet Gynaecol. 1980;87:408-12.
16. De Ligny WR, Kerkhof MH, Ruiz-Zapata AM. Regenerative medicine as a therapeutic option for fecal incontinence: A systematic review of preclinical and clinical studies. Am J Obstet Gynecol. 2019;220:142-54.e2.
17. DeLancey JO, Toglia MR, Perucchini D. Internal and External Anal Sphincter Anatomy as it Relates to Midline Obstetric Lacerations. Obstet Gynecol. 1997;90:924-7.
18. Dietz HP. Exoanal imaging of the anal sphincters. J Ultrasound Med. 2018;37:263-80.
19. Dobben AC, Terra MP, Slors JFM, Deutekom M, Gerhards MF, Beets-Tan RG, et al. Comparison of endoanal MRI and endoanal ultra-sonography in the depiction of external anal sphincter defects in fecal incontinent patients. Radiology. 2007;242:463-71.
20. Faltin DL, Boulvain M, Irion O, Bretones S, Stan C, Weil A. Diagnosis of anal sphincter tears by postpartum endosonography to predict fecal incontinence. Obstet Gynecol. 2000;95:643-7.
21. Farrell SA, Flowerdew G, Gilmour D, Turnbull GK, Schmidt MH, Baskett TF, et al. Overlapping compared with end-to-end repair of complete third-degree or fourth-degree obstetric tears: Three-year follow-up of a randomized controlled trial. Obstet Gynecol. 2012;120:803.

22. Fatakia FT, Subramaniam N, Bienkiewicz J, Friedman T, Dietz HP. How repeatable is assessment of external anal sphincter trauma by exoanal 4D ultrasound? Ultrasound Obstet Gynecol. 2019;53:836-40.
23. Fattorini E, Brusa T, Gingert C, Hieber SE, Leung V, Osmani B, et al. Artificial Muscle Devices: Innovations and Prospects for FI Treatment. Ann Biomed Eng. 2016;44:1355-69.
24. Fenner DE, Genberg B, Brahma P, Marek L, DeLancey JO. Fecal and urinary incontinence after vaginal delivery with anal sphincter disruption in an obstetrics unit in the United States. Am J Obstet Gynecol. 2003;189:1543-9.
25. Fernando RJ, Sultan AH, Freeman RM, Williams AA, Adams EJ. The Management of Third- and Fourth-Degree Perineal Tears (Green-Top Guideline No. 29). London, UK: Royal College of Obstetricians and Gynaecologists; 2015.
26. Fernando RJ, Sultan AH, Kettle C, Thakar R. Methods of repair for obstetric anal sphincter injury. Cochrane Database Syst Rev. 2013:CD002866.
27. Fowler G, Adams E, Bolderson J, Hosker G, Lowe D, Richmond D, et al. Liverpool Ultrasound Pictorial Chart: The development of a new method of documenting anal sphincter injury diagnosed by endoanal ultrasound. BJOG Int J Obstet Gynaecol. 2008;115:767-72.
28. García-Mejido JA, Palomino LG, Palacín AF, Sainz-Bueno JA. Applicability of 3/4D transperineal ultrasound for the diagnosis of anal sphincter injury during the immediate postpartum. Cir Cir (Engl. Ed.). 2017;85:80-6.
29. Gurol-Urganci I, Cromwell DA, Edozien LC, Mahmood TA, Adams EJ, Richmond DH, et al. Third- and fourth-degree perineal tears among primiparous women in England between 2000 and 2012: Time trends and risk factors. BJOG Int J Obstet Gynaecol. 2013;120:1516-25.
30. Harvey MA, Pierce M, Walter JE, Chou Q, Diamond P, Epp A, et al. Obstetrical Anal Sphincter Injuries (OASIS): Prevention, Recognition, and Repair. J Obstet Gynaecol Can. 2015;37:1131-48.
31. Hetzer FH, Andreisek G, Tsagari C, Sahrbacher U, Weishaupt M. MR Defecography in patients with fecal incontinence: Imaging findings and their effect on surgical management 1. Radiology. 2006;240:449-57.
32. Huang WC, Yang SH, Yang JM. Three-dimensional transperineal sonographic characteristics of the anal sphincter complex in nulliparous women. Ultrasound Obstet. Gynecol. 2007;30:210-20.
33. Hull T, Giese C, Wexner SD, Mellgren A, Devroede G, Madoff RD, et al. Long-term Durability of Sacral Nerve Stimulation Therapy for Chronic Fecal Incontinence. Dis. Colon Rectum. 2013;56:234-45.
34. Jha S, Parker V. Risk factors for recurrent obstetric anal sphincter injury (rOASI): A systematic review and meta-analysis. Int Urogynecol J. 2016;27:849-57.
35. Jiang HH, Song QX, Gill BC, Balog BM, Juarez R, Cruz Y, et al. Electrical stimulation of the pudendal nerve promotes neuroregeneration and functional recovery from stress urinary incontinence in a rat model. Am J Physiol Physiol. 2018;315:F1555-64.
36. Jorge JM, Wexner SD. Etiology and management of fecal in- continence. Dis Colon Rectum. 1993;36:77-97.
37. Kaiser AM, Orangio GR, Zutshi M, Alva S, Hull TL, Marcello PW, et al. Current status: New technologies for the treatment of patients with fecal incontinence. Surg Endosc. 2014;28:2277-301.

38. Kapoor DS, Thakar R, Sultan AH. Obstetric anal sphincter injuries: Review of anatomical factors and modifiable second stage interventions. Int Urogynecol J. 2015;26:1725-34.
39. Keag OE, Norman JE, Stock SJ. Long-term risks and benefits associated with cesarean delivery for mother, baby, and subsequent pregnancies: Systematic review and meta-analysis. PLoS Med. 2018;15:e1002494.
40. Kettle C, Tohill S. Perineal care. BMJ Clin Évid. 2008;2008:1401.
41. Kirss J, Huhtinen H, Niskanen E, Ruohonen J, Kallio-Packalen M, Victorzon S, et al. Comparison of 3D endoanal ultrasound and external phased array magnetic resonance imaging in the diagnosis of obstetric anal sphincter injuries. Eur Radiol. 2019;29:5717-22.
42. Krissi H, Aviram A, Hiersch L, Ashwal E, Eitan R, Peled Y. Structured hands-on workshop decreases the over-detection rate of obstetrical anal sphincter injuries. Int J Color Dis. 2015;31:45-50.
43. Lowder JL, Burrows LJ, Krohn MA, Weber AM. Risk factors for primary and subsequent anal sphincter lacerations: A comparison of cohorts by parity and prior mode of delivery. Am J Obstet Gynecol. 2007;196:344.e1-344.e5.
44. Maeda Y, Laurberg S, Norton C. Perianal injectable bulking agents as treatment for faecal incontinence in adults. Cochrane Database Syst. Rev. 2013: CD007959.
45. Magro PMH, Saenz EV, Zavala MJ, Munro RDS, Ramírez JLR. Endoanal sonography in assessment of fecal incontinence following obstetric trauma. Ultrasound Obstet Gynecol. 2003;22:616-21.
46. Milsom I, Altman D, Cartwright R, Lapitan MC, Nelson R, Sillén U, Tikkanen K. Epidemiology of Urinary Incontinence (UI) and other Lower Urinary Tract Symptoms (LUTS), Pelvic Organ Prolapse (POP) and Anal (AI) Incontinence. In: Abrams P, Cardozo L, Kouhry S, Wein A (eds). Incontinence, 5th edition. Paris, France: Health Publications Ltd.; 2013. pp. 15-107.
47. Młyńczak M, Rosoł M, Spinelli A, Dziki A, Wlazlak E, Surkont G, et al. Obstetric Anal Sphincter Injury Detection Using Impedance Spectroscopy with the ONIRY Probe. Appl Sci. 2021;11:63761.
48. Nordenstam J, Mellgren A, Altman D, López A, Johansson C, Anzén B, et al. Immediate or delayed repair of obstetric anal sphincter tears-a randomised controlled trial. BJOG Int J Obstet Gynaecol. 2008;115:857-65.
49. Oakley SH, Ghodsi VC, Crisp CC, Estanol MV, Westermann LB, Novicki KM, et al. Impact of Pelvic Floor Physical Therapy on Quality of Life and Function After Obstetric Anal Sphincter Injury: A Randomized Controlled Trial. Female Pelvic Med Reconstr Surg. 2016;22:205-13.
50. Ohannessen HH, Wibe A, Stordahl A, Sandvik L, Mørkved S. Do pelvic floor muscle exercises reduce postpartum anal incontinence? A randomised controlled trial. BJOG Int J Obstet Gynaecol. 2016;124:686-94.
51. Pannu HK, Javitt MC, Glanc P, Bhosale PR, Harisinghani MG, Khati NJ, et al. ACR Appropriateness Criteria Pelvic Floor Dysfunction. J Am Coll Radiol. 2015;12:134-42.
52. Paquette IM, Varma MG, Kaiser AM, Steele SR, Rafferty JF. The American Society of Colon and Rectal Surgeons' Clinical Practice Guideline for the Treatment of Fecal Incontinence. Dis Colon Rectum. 2015;58:623-36.

53. Parmar N, Kumar L, Emmanuel A, Day RM. Prospective regenerative medicine therapies for obstetric trauma-induced fecal incontinence. Regen Med. 2014;9:831-40.
54. Pescatori M, Anastasio G, Bottini C, Mentasti A. New grading and scoring for anal incontinence. Dis Colon Rectum. 1992;35:482-7.
55. Rojas RAG, Kamisan Atan I, Shek KL, Dietz HP. Anal sphincter trauma and anal incontinence in urogynecological patients. Ultrasound Obstet Gynecol. 2015;46:363-6.
56. Rojas RAG, Salvesen KÅ, Volløyhaug I. Anal sphincter defects and fecal incontinence 15–24 years after first delivery: A cross-sectional study; Ultrasound Obstet Gynecol. 2018;51:677-83.
57. Rojas RAG, Shek KL, Langer SM, Dietz HP. The prevalence of anal sphincter injury in primiparous women. Ultrasound Obstet Gynecol. 2013;42:461-6.
58. Ruiz NS, Kaiser AM. Fecal incontinence—Challenges and solutions. World J Gastroenterol. 2017;23:11-24.
59. Salvador JC, Coutinho MP, Venâncio JM, Viamonte B. Dynamic magnetic resonance imaging of the female pelvic floor—A pictorial review. Insights Imaging. 2019;10:1-16.
60. Schwandner T, Hemmelmann C, Heimerl T, Kierer W, Kolbert G, Vonthein R, et al. Triple-Target Treatment Versus Low-Frequency Electrostimulation for Anal Incontinence. Dtsch. Aerzteblatt Online. 2011;108:653.
61. Simillis C, Lal N, Pellino G, Baird D, Nikolaou S, Kontovounisios C, et al. A systematic review and network meta-analysis comparing treatments for faecal incontinence. Int J Surg. 2019;66:37-47.
62. Snooks S, Swash M, Setchell M, Henry M. Injury to innervation of pelvic floor sphincter musculature in childbirth. Lancet. 1984;2:546-50.
63. Stock L, Basham E, Gossett D, Lewicky-Gaupp C. Factors associated with wound complications in women with obstetric anal sphincter injuries (OASIS) Am J Obstet Gynecol. 2013;208:327.e1-327.e6.
64. Stuart A, Ignell C, Örnö A. Comparison of transperineal and endoanal ultrasound in detecting residual obstetric anal sphincter injury. Acta Obstet Gynecol Scand. 2019;98:1624-31.
65. Sultan AH, Kamm MA, Hudson CN, Bartram CI. Third degree obstetric anal sphincter tears: Risk factors and outcome of primary repair. BMJ. 1994;308: 887-91.
66. Sultan AH, Monga AK, Kumar D, Stanton SL. Primary repair of obstetric anal sphincter rupture using the overlap technique. BJOG Int J Obstet Gynaecol. 1999;106:318-23.
67. Sultan AH. Obstetric perineal injury and anal incontinence. Clin. Risk. 1999;5:193-6.
68. Taithongchai A, van Gruting IM, Volløyhaug I, Arendsen LP, Sultan AH, Thakar R. Comparing the diagnostic accuracy of 3 ultrasound modalities for diagnosing obstetric anal sphincter injuries. Am J Obstet Gynecol. 2019;221:134. e1-134.e9.
69. Tan EK, Vaizey C, Cornish J, Darzi A, Tekkis PP. Surgical strategies for faecal incontinence-a decision analysis between dynamic graciloplasty, artificial bowel sphincter and end stoma. Colorectal Dis. 2008;10:577-86.

70. Tetzschner T, Sorensen M, Lose G, Christiansen J. Anal and urinary incontinence in women with obstetric anal sphincter rupture. BJOG Int J Obstet Gynaecol. 1996;103:1034-40.
71. Thaha MA, Abukar AA, Thin NN, Ramsanahie A, Knowles CH. Sacral nerve stimulation for faecal incontinence and constipation in adults. Cochrane Database Syst Rev. 2015:CD004464.
72. Thin NN, Horrocks EJ, Hotouras A, Palit S, Thaha MA, Chan CLH, et al. Systematic review of the clinical effectiveness of neuromodulation in the treatment of faecal incontinence. BJS. 2013;100:1430-47.
73. Thomas GP, Gould LE, Casunuran F, Kumar DA. A retrospective review of 1495 patients with obstetric anal sphincter injuries referred for assessment of function and endoanal ultrasonography. Int J Color Dis. 2017;32:1321-5.
74. Uustal Fornell EK, Berg G, Hallbook O, Matthiesen LS, Sjodahal R. Clinical consequence of anal sphincter rupture during vaginal delivery. J Am Coll Surg. 1996;183:553-8.
75. Vaizey CJ, Carapeti E, Cahill JA, Kamm MA. Prospective comparison of fecal incontinence grading systems. Gut. 1999;44:77-80.
76. Valsky DV, Cohen SM, Lipschuetz M, Hochner-Celnikier D, Yagel S. Three-dimensional transperineal ultrasound findings associated with anal incontinence after intrapartum sphincter tears in primiparous women. Ultrasound Obstet Gynecol. 2011;39:83-90.
77. Valsky DV, Messing B, Petkova R, Savchev S, Rosenak D, Hochner-Celnikier D, et al. Postpartum evaluation of the anal sphincter by transperineal three-dimensional ultrasound in primiparous women after vaginal delivery and following surgical repair of third-degree tears by the overlapping technique. Ultrasound Obstet Gynecol. 2007;29:195-204.
78. Van Koughnett JAM, da Silva G. Anorectal physiology and testing. Gastroenterol Clin N Am. 2013;42:713-28.
79. Wallace SL, Miller LD, Mishra K. Pelvic floor physical therapy in the treatment of pelvic floor dysfunction in women. Curr Opin Obstet Gynecol. 2019;31: 485-93.
80. Walsh KA, Grivell RM. Use of endoanal ultrasound for reducing the risk of complications related to anal sphincter injury after vaginal birth. Cochrane Database Syst Rev. 2015;10:CD010826.
81. West RL, Dwarkasing S, Briel JW, Hansen BE, Hussain SM, Schouten WR, et al. Can 3D endoanal ultrasonography detect external anal sphincter atrophy? A comparison with endoanal. MRI Int J Colorectal Dis. 2005;20:328-33.
82. Wilson D, Dornan J, Milsom I, Freeman R. UR-CHOICE: Can we provide mothers-to-be with information about the risk of future pelvic floor dysfunction? Int Urogynecol J. 2014;25:1449-52.

9 CHAPTER

Complications of Vaginal Hysterectomy

Anil Sakhare, Juhi Agarwal

INTRODUCTION

Traditionally, vaginal hysterectomy has been the hallmark procedure defining a gynecologic surgeon. Vaginal hysterectomy (VH) is a commonly performed gynecological surgery indicated for benign uterine conditions such as prolapse, fibroids, abnormal uterine bleeding, and chronic pelvic pain (for reasons of Chronic PID). Compared with abdominal and laparoscopic hysterectomy, the vaginal route is often preferred due to its shorter hospital stay, reduced postoperative pain, fewer wound complications, and faster recovery. Despite these advantages, vaginal hysterectomy is not free from complications. Understanding the potential intraoperative and postoperative complications is essential for patient counselling, surgical planning, and minimizing morbidity. Vaginal Hysterectomy offers reduced operating times and faster recovery in comparison to alternative techniques, with comparable complication rates. If VH is at a survival- revival stage, it also means if surgeons are doing it as a learning- procedure, more complications are likely. But we feel some complications must be peculiar to each procedure as in LH some complications are purely because of energy sources used. If use of energy sources in VH are avoided, pattern of complications would differ. This article discusses the major and minor complications associated with vaginal hysterectomy, their risk factors, clinical manifestations, preventive strategies, and management options. This article gives the links of video presentation of few surgical techniques which will help the readers to understand the technical aspect of the procedure which will help to minimize the complications while performing vaginal hysterectomy.

INTRAOPERATIVE COMPLICATIONS

Hemorrhage

Hemorrhage is among the most common and serious intraoperative complications of VH. It may arise from excessive traction on the uterine vessels, injury during vaginal wall dissection, or inadequate hemostasis. Risk factors include enlarged uterus, dense pelvic adhesions, previous pelvic surgeries, and coagulopathies. Excessive bleeding may require conversion to an abdominal procedure, blood transfusion, or ligation of pelvic vessels. Preventive steps include careful preoperative evaluation, efficient surgical technique, appropriate use of electrosurgery.

Bladder Injury

Bladder injury occurs in 0.5–1% of vaginal hysterectomy cases and is often related to difficult dissection in patients with previous cesarean deliveries or pelvic inflammatory disease. Bladder injury increases with risk factors like prior pelvic surgeries and concomitant bladder surgeries. Bladder injury during vaginal hysterectomy has been variously reported between 0.5 and 1.6%. Unger, reported an incidence of 2.8% in the past LSCS group versus 1.6% in those without LSCS. Sheth reported an exceptionally low incidence of bladder injury of 0.1%. The bladder is most vulnerable during the anterior colpotomy. There are various techniques described to tackle cesarean section scar while opening anterior pouch. Entering through Shirish Seth space is the most followed method where there is less adhesions and less vascularity in this space. Another method which author follows is the traction by allies forceps on cervix and counter traction by sims speculum over anterior vaginal wall and sharp dissection over the scar *(VDO of this method can be seen on the following link-https://youtu.be/Ts4CpkUxmtM)*. If recognized intraoperatively, bladder injury should be repaired immediately with layered closure and postoperative catheterization for 7–14 days. Undetected injuries may later present as urinary leakage or vesicovaginal fistula.

Ureteric Injury

Though less common in vaginal hysterectomy compared with abdominal or laparoscopic routes, ureteric injury can occur, especially during clamping of the cardinal and uterosacral ligaments. The ureter may be kinked, ligated, or inadvertently transected. Clinical suspicion should arise in cases of excessive bleeding, distorted anatomy, or large pelvic masses. Preventive strategies include careful identification of anatomical landmarks and avoiding blind clamping. Intraoperative cystoscopy with dye testing may help confirm ureteric patency. Surgeon can stay away from ureters during surgery just by pulling the uterus downward and in opposite direction which keep surgical field away from ureter. *(VDO of this technique can be seen on following link-https://youtu.be/T6jCv-D33oY)*. Most commonly ureter get caught in the clamp or suture when the uterosacral and Mackenrodt's ligament have to religate for achieving hemostasis. This is very common in cases of adenomyosis where the ligaments are shortened and stout. Special care should be taken when surgeon is using energy devices.

Rectal Injury

Rectal injury is uncommon but may occur in cases with rectocele, severe endometriosis, or dense adhesions. A small rectal perforation, if detected, should be repaired immediately with layered closure. Failure to recognize the injury may lead to pelvic abscess, peritonitis, or rectovaginal fistula.

Bowel Injury

Injury to small or large intestine is rare during vaginal hysterectomy. It usually occurs when there is prolapsing bowel, adhesions from prior surgeries, or inadvertent entry into the peritoneal cavity. Prompt recognition and repair are crucial to prevent postoperative sepsis or bowel obstruction. An innovative technique called as cervical colpotomy can minimizes the bowl injury in cases with suspected adhesions in pouch of Douglas *(VDO of this procedure can be seen on following link https://youtu.be/CyzYbC-XaK0).*

Anesthetic Complications

Like any surgical procedure, VH may be associated with anesthetic complications such as hypotension, allergic reactions, respiratory depression, or cardiac events. These risks are minimized through preoperative assessment, intraoperative monitoring, and skilled anesthetic management.

POSTOPERATIVE COMPLICATIONS

Infection

Postoperative infections are among the most frequent complications after vaginal hysterectomy.

Vaginal Cuff Infection

This includes cellulitis or abscess formation at the surgical site. The patients with vault cellulitis usually present with fever, which is the earliest sign of infection. Toglia et al., found in their study that 69% of women with postoperative pelvic collection experienced febrile morbidity compared to 12% with no collection. The other symptoms of vault cellulitis is foul smelling discharge which may be scanty or profuse and sometimes may be blood tinged. Pain and tenderness in the pelvic area may be experienced due to the infection. Some patients may also present with swelling and redness in the vaginal vault area. In a study done in Ukraine, a total of 12.6% of women after hysterectomy had vaginal cuff infections. Of these cases, 15.5% after vaginal hysterectomy were identified. Symptoms include fever, pelvic pain, and purulent discharge. Treatment involves antibiotics and, in some cases, surgical drainage.

Urinary Tract Infection

Urinary tract infections (UTIs) are common due to catheterization and proximity to the urethra. Adequate catheter care, early removal, and hydration help reduce the risk.

Pelvic Abscess

Although rare, pelvic abscess may develop due to unrecognized bowel injury or deep infection. Management may require intravenous antibiotics and radiologically guided drainage. Few nonresponding cases may require exploration by abdominal route. We consider opening the vault, if we are sure abscess is not because of bowel injury and is just above the vault on TVS.

Hemorrhage and Hematoma

Postoperative hemorrhage may occur due to slippage of ligatures, infection, or inadequate hemostasis. Vaginal vault hematomas typically present with pelvic pain, fullness, and fever. Small hematomas may resolve spontaneously, while large ones more than 5 cm require drainage. Hematomas are mainly formed in the dead space between the peritoneum and vaginal vault. Proper approximation of these will help to prevent most of the hematomas *(VDO of this procedure can be seen on following link https://youtu.be/UQ1AU_ogKtk).*

Urinary Complications

Urinary Retention

Transient retention is relatively common due to postoperative pain, edema, or spinal anesthesia. Intermittent catheterization or short-term indwelling catheter use helps manage this condition.

Fistula Formation

Vesicovaginal or ureterovaginal fistula may develop secondary to unrecognized intraoperative injury. Patients present with continuous urinary leakage. Clamp, suture ligation, partial or total primary transection, angulation, avulsion, or ischemic necrosis following electrocoagulation are examples of mechanisms that can cause ureter damage during surgical procedures. Treatment may involve prolonged catheterization or surgical repair. Severe ureteral strictures, urogenital fistulas, and renal insufficiency caused by ureteral injuries necessitate more comprehensive reconstructive surgery.

Bowel Complications

Constipation and Ileus

Postoperative constipation is common due to anesthesia, opioids, and decreased mobility. Ileus may present with abdominal distension, nausea, and vomiting. Prevention includes adequate hydration, early mobilization, stool softeners, and minimizing opioid use.

Rectovaginal Fistula

A rare complication often resulting from unrecognized rectal injury or infection. It causes passage of feces or gas through the vagina. Surgical repair is usually required.

Thromboembolic Events

Deep vein thrombosis (DVT) and pulmonary embolism (PE) are serious postoperative complications, though relatively uncommon due to early mobilization and minimally invasive nature of VH. High-risk patients (obesity, advanced age, malignancy, smoking, thrombophilia) may require prophylactic anticoagulants and compression devices.

Vaginal Vault Prolapse

Vaginal vault prolapse can occur months or years after hysterectomy due to inadequate support of the pelvic floor. It is more common in patients with preexisting pelvic organ prolapse. Preventive measures include proper reattachment of the uterosacral or cardinal ligaments during surgery. We found McCall culdoplasty is best and simple procedure for vault prolapse prevention especially in cases of prolapse. Treatment options include pelvic floor exercises, pessary use, or surgical repair.

Sexual Dysfunction

Some women may experience dyspareunia, decreased libido, or vaginal dryness following hysterectomy. These symptoms may be due to scar formation, hormonal changes, psychological factors, or vaginal cuff shortening. Appropriate counselling, lubricants, pelvic physiotherapy, and hormone therapy (if indicated) can help.

Chronic Pelvic Pain

Persistent pelvic pain after VH may result from nerve entrapment especially genitofemoral nerve entrapment, pelvic floor dysfunction, infection, or adhesions. A thorough evaluation is required to identify the underlying cause. Management may involve analgesics, physiotherapy, treatment of infection, or surgical intervention.

Psychological and Emotional Effects

Although vaginal hysterectomy is performed for medical reasons, it can lead to emotional distress, feelings of loss, or anxiety in some patients. Preoperative counselling and postoperative psychological support are important components of care.

FACTORS INFLUENCING COMPLICATION RATES

Several factors influence the risk of complications in vaginal hysterectomy:

- *Patient-related factors:* Age, obesity, parity, comorbidities (diabetes, hypertension), history of pelvic surgery, connective tissue disorders.
- *Uterine size:* Larger uteri increase the difficulty of dissection.
- *Pelvic adhesions:* From endometriosis, pelvic inflammatory disease.
- *Surgeon experience:* Skill and familiarity with vaginal techniques significantly reduce complication rates.
- *Intraoperative findings:* Abnormal anatomy or unexpected bleeding increase risks.

A careful preoperative evaluation—including pelvic examination, imaging when necessary, and review of medical history—helps determine suitability for vaginal hysterectomy and minimizes complications.

PREVENTION AND RISK REDUCTION

Prevention of complications involves a combination of proper patient selection, skilled surgical technique, and comprehensive perioperative care.

Preoperative Measures

- Detailed history and physical examination
- Identification of risk factors such as anemia, diabetes, or infections
- Prophylactic antibiotics
- Bowel and bladder preparation if indicated
- Counseling regarding expectations and possible complications

Intraoperative Measures

- Adequate exposure and lighting
- Gentle tissue handling
- Clear identification of bladder, rectum, and ureters
- Use of appropriate instruments and energy sources
- Cystoscopy when risk of ureteric injury is high

Postoperative Care

- Early ambulation
- Pain control with minimal opioid use

- Adequate hydration and bowel management
- Monitoring of vital signs and wound healing
- Follow-up visits to assess recovery

CONCLUSION

Vaginal hysterectomy is a safe and effective surgical procedure with significant advantages over abdominal routes. However, like any operative intervention, it carries the potential for complications—both intraoperative and postoperative. Awareness of these complications, along with risk factors and preventative strategies, enables the surgeon to minimize morbidity and ensure better patient outcomes. Proper preoperative evaluation, meticulous surgical technique, and postoperative monitoring form the cornerstone of safe vaginal hysterectomy practice. With skilled hands and comprehensive care, most complications can be avoided or effectively managed, ensuring a high success rate and patient satisfaction.

SUGGESTED READING

1. American College of Obstetricians and Gynecologists. Practice Bulletin No. 205: Hysterectomy for benign conditions. Washington (DC): ACOG; 2020.
2. Harmanli O, Gentzler CK, Byun S, Dandolu V. Intraoperative complications of vaginal hysterectomy. Int Urogynecol J. 2011;22(12):1481-5.
3. Johnson N, Barlow D, Lethaby A. Surgical approach to hysterectomy for benign gynaecological disease. Cochrane Database Syst Rev. 2006;(2):CD003677.
4. Kovac SR. Vaginal hysterectomy: rationale and surgical approach. Obstet Gynecol. 2004;103(6):1321-5.
5. Muzii L, Basile S, Bellati F, Zullo MA, Manci N, Panici PB. The role of vaginal hysterectomy. Best Pract Res Clin Obstet Gynaecol. 2007;21(2):231-41.
6. Oliva R, Forgione A, Akladios C, Querleu D, Mastrovito S, Pavone M, et al. Is vaginal hysterectomy outdated? A systematic overview of reviews with future perspectives. J Gynecol Obstet Hum Reprod. 2025;54(7):102968.
7. Ratajczak JM, Hladun T, Orchel G. Latrogenic ureterovaginal fistula after laparoscopic hysterectomy: a case report. Prz Menopauzalny. 2021;20:48-51.
8. Salmanov AG, Vitiuk AD, Hrynchuk SY, Bober AS, Hrynchuk OB, Berestooy OA, et al. Vaginal cuff infection after hysterectomy in Ukraine. Wiad Lek. 2021;74:196-201.
9. Sheth SS. The scope of vaginal hysterectomy. Eur J Obstet Gynecol Reprod Biol. 2004;115(2):224-30.
10. Toglia MR, Pearlman MD. Pelvic fluid collections following hysterectomy and their relation to febrile morbidity. Obstet Gynecol 1994;83:766-70.
11. Unger JB, Meeks GR. Vaginal hysterectomy in women with history of previous cesarean delivery. Am J Obstet Gynecol. 1998;179(6):1473-578.

10 CHAPTER

Debulking Techniques During Vaginal Hysterectomy

Mukesh Rathi

INTRODUCTION

Historically, debulking or volume reduction techniques have been described way back in late 19th and mid-20th century by various gynecological surgeons, like Amussat, Czerny, Muller, Pryor, Lash, and many others. The aim basically was to remove the uterus by the least invasive, vaginal route

INDICATIONS FOR DEBULKING

Whenever the size or the mobility of the uterus are a hinderance for sheering of the parametrial attachments, or delivery of the fibroid or uterus, by way of limitation of space or descent, then one needs to adopt the debulking techniques.

Principles of Debulking

Principle is gradual volume reduction so that the big size uterus/fibroids, adnexal mass can be delivered out or induce the giveaway of the uterine muscular wall, to facilitate gentle delivery.

CRITERIA FOR DECIDING THE APPROACH

- *Clinical examination:* Assessment of the laxity of vagina, size, mobility, descent of the uterus, the number and location of the fibroids.
- Added factors like previous LSCS or any uterine surgeries
- USG for volume of the uterus, mapping the fibroids, associated adnexal pathology
- Examination under anesthesia for mobility, size, and descent
- Surgeon's experience backed up by the patient's willingness

CONTRAINDICATIONS

- Malignancy must be ruled out
- When the transverse axis of the uterus is more than the longitudinal axis (banyan tree appearance) **(Fig. 1)**.

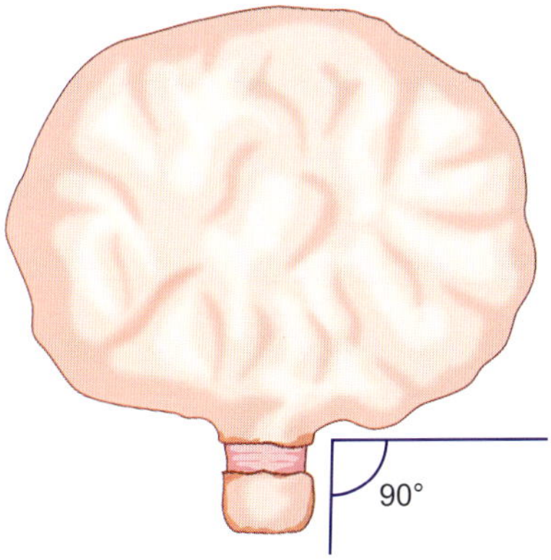

Fig. 1: Transverse axis more than the longitudinal axis.

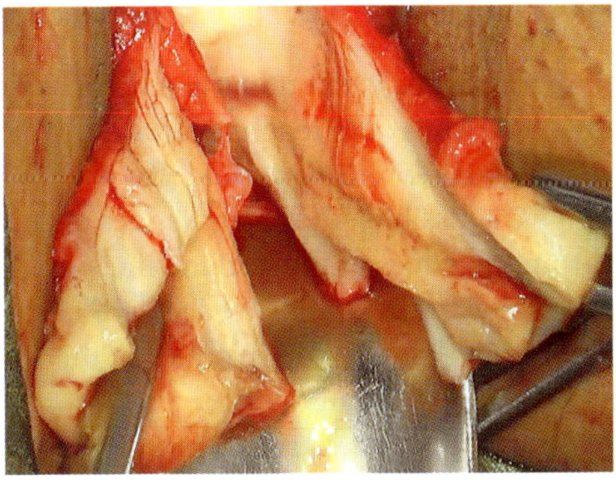

Fig. 2: Bisection.

PRECAUTIONS

- Bladder should be empty/catheterized
- Bladder and rectum secured under the respective anterior and posterior retractors.
  - Avoid cluttering of the instruments or retractors
  - Morcellation should begin only after securing the uterine vascular bundle and under vision
  - Should know when to abandon

VARIOUS TECHNIQUES OF DEBULKING

- *Bisection/hemisection* ***(Fig. 2)****:* After the uterine vascular bundle is secured, steady traction is applied on the uterus and an incision in taken right from the cervix, vertically upwards, through the anterior and posterior wall. This induces give away of the myometrial muscle fibers and the uterus descends. Works well for up to 10–12 weeks size uterus.

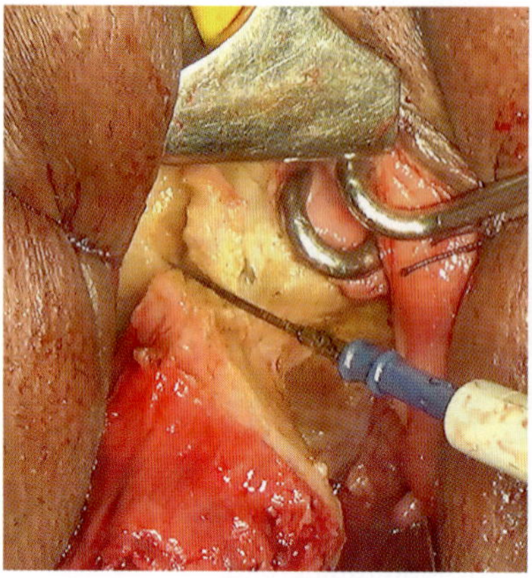

Fig. 3: Wedge morcellation.

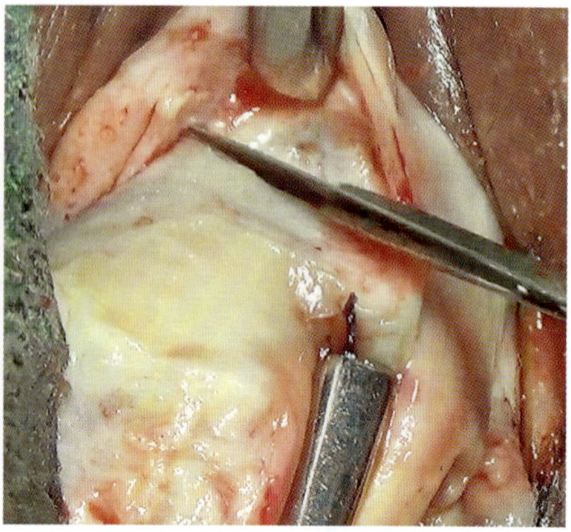

Fig. 4: Coring Lash and Lash.

- *Transection:* Here the uterus is cut transversely, so as to give more space to tackle the adnexal tissues or to reach the fibroid.
- *Pryor's technique (Anterior wedge morcellation)* ***(Fig. 3)****:* Uterus is bisected till as high as possible. After that, wedges of the uterine tissue are cut, anteriorly from the edges of the midline incision. The everted edges are further pulled down and similar wedges are cut from the part that descends, till the fundus is reached. Myomas on the way are enucleated. Works well when the POD is obliterated.
- *Anteroposterior Wedge resection:* Cut the chunks of myometrium through the entire wall using the tenaculum or myoma screws, with the apex of the wedge digging into the substance of the uterine tissue, creating a sort of tunnel so that the walls collapse on each other, giving space for further progression
- *Lash's technique (Coring)* ***(Fig. 4)****:* Well suited for elongated globular uteri or when subpubic angle is narrow. Circumferential incisions are taken serially on the myometrium, just below the serosa. This causes the inversion of serosa and myometrium above. Similar serial incisions are taken to deliver the uterus in a process like peeling a banana.

DEBULKING OF THE BENIGN ADNEXAL CYSTIC MASSES (FIG. 5)

After the uterus is removed, traction is applied in the downward and outward direction on the cornual pedicle to bring the cyst in view & a small pack is pushed behind the cyst. Depending upon the size, a Veress needle or a 5 mm laparoscopic trocar-cannula is pushed in the cyst. Suction is applied through the needle or a suction cannula, that drains the entire cyst. The cyst drops into the field of surgery cystectomy or oophorectomy can be done as per the need.

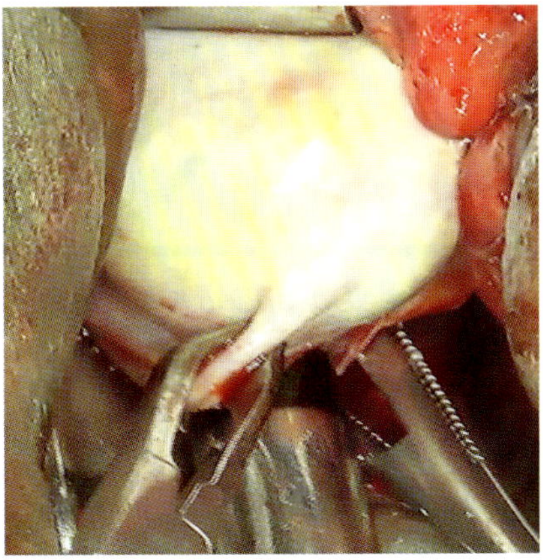

Fig. 5: Suction aspiration of big dermoid.

SUGGESTED READING

1. Dubuisson J, Veit-Rubin N. Uterine volume and vaginal hysterectomy: Interest and limits of uterine morcellation. Gynecol Obstet Fertil. 2016;44(3): 175-80.
2. Lash AF. A method of reducing the size of the uterus in vaginal hysterectomy. Am J Obstet Gynaecol. 1941;42:452.
3. Nazah I, Robin F. Comparison between bisection/morcellation and myometrial coring for reducing large uteriduring Vaginal hysterectomy or LAVH: Results of a randomized prospective study. Acta Obstet Gynaecol Scand. 2003;82: 1037-42.
4. Quinlan D. Vaginal hysterectomy in enlarged uterus - a report of 85 cases. J Obstet Gynaecol Can. 2010;32:980-3.
5. Sahen Y. Vaginal hysterectomy and oopherectomy in women with 12–20 weeks size uterus: Acta Obstet Gynaecol Scand. 2007;86:1359-69.
6. Sheth SS. Adnexectomy for benign pathology at vaginal hysterectomy without laparoscopic assistance. Br J Obstet Gynaecol. 2002;109:1401-5.
7. Sheth SS. Broad ligament myomectomy at vaginal hysterectomy without laparoscopic assistance. J Gynaecol Surg. 2007;23:133-42.
8. Sheth SS. Preoperative sonographic estimation of uterine volume: an aid to determine the route of hysterectomy. J Gynaecol Surg. 2002:18:13-22.
9. Wasson M, Butler K, Magtibay P, Temkit M, Magrina J. Prognostic Factors for Morcellation During Vaginal Hysterectomy. Obstet Gynecol. 2016;127(4): 752-7.
10. Wasson MN, Butler KA, Temkit M, Magrina JF. Necessity of Morcellation at Time of Vaginal Hysterectomy. J Minim Invasive Gynecol. 2015;22(6S):S12.

11 CHAPTER

Sacrospinous Fixation

Rajshree Dayanand Katke, Nidhi Sharma Chauhann

INTRODUCTION

In women with vault prolapse, massive vaginal eversion and procidentia, Sacrospinous fixation has become the favored surgery of choice. Sacrospinous colpopexy, also known as Sacrospinous fixation, was introduced way back in 1971 by Randall and Nichols.

Maintenance of the apical support is very important in the treatment of prolapse. Sacrospinous fixation surgery provides the Apical support.

A good knowledge of the anatomy of the attachments and relations of the Sacrospinous ligament is crucial to ensure a safe outcome. The upper third of the vagina is suspended from the pelvic walls by the vertical fibers of the paracolpium. The sacrospinous and the uterosacral ligament fixation add to the level 1 support.

The Pudendal nerve and vessels lie behind the sacrospinous ligament. They lie medially and inferiorly in relation to the ischial spine. The inferior gluteal artery also lies behind the sacrospinous ligament.

Sacrospinous fixation can be done after a vaginal hysterectomy as a prophylactic measure to prevent future vault prolapse. Sacrospinous colpopexy is also done in cases of vault prolapse which may develop after a vaginal, abdominal or laparoscopic hysterectomy, even though the incidence is very less.

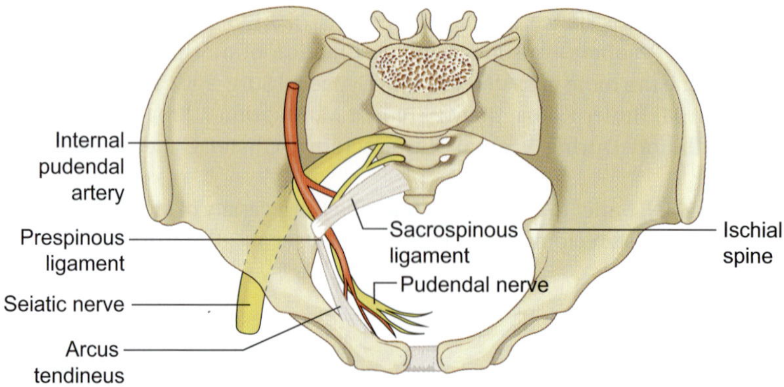

Fig. 1: Anatomy of the sacrospinous ligament.

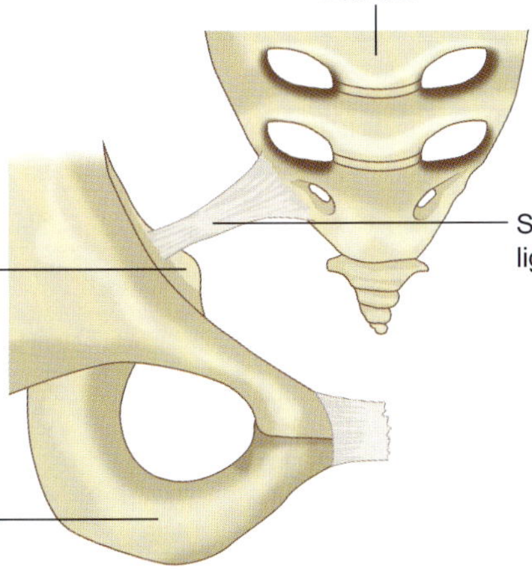

Fig. 2: Anatomical relation of the sacrospinous ligament to the ischial spine.

Surgical repair of vault prolapse can be done via the abdominal route or the vaginal route. Abdominal sacro colpopexy is done via Laparoscopy. The Sacrospinous fixation is done via the vaginal route. This approach is less invasive than the abdominal approach. There is lesser postoperative pain and faster return to work after the Sacrospinous fixation.

OPERATIVE TECHNIQUE

The approach to doing a sacrospinous fixation is by the vaginal route.

Various operative techniques have been described and used for the correction of the apical prolapse.

The surgery is done under general anesthesia in a lithotomy position. Vaginal hysterectomy is done as initially followed by fixation of the sacrospinous ligament. The rectovaginal space is exposed by giving longitudinal incision in the posterior vaginal wall. The pararectal space is then opened on the right side. The ligament is usually suspended on the patient's right side because the traction of the rectum is easier and for most surgeons who are right handed, it is technically easier to pass the suture. Using the ischial spine as the landmark, the sacrospinous ligament is palpated. A long needle holder (12 inch) is used to place the suture starting from the superior border of the ligament in an upside-down direction. The suture is placed 2 cm medial to the ischial spine to prevent an injury to the pudendal nerve and internal pudendal vessels. The suture is retrieved as a loop and is then decided to establish two sutures. The sutures are then places through the full thickness of vaginal muscularis at the point of the new vaginal apex, once the enterocele closure and anterior colporrhaphy have been done. The sutures of the sacrospinous ligament are now tied once the vaginal cuff is closed. This brings the sacrospinous ligament in

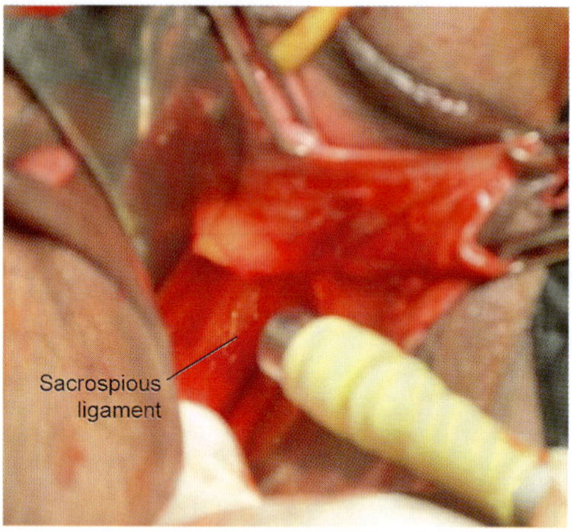

Fig. 3: Sacrospinous ligament vaginally.
Courtesy: Dr Rajshree Dayanand Katke

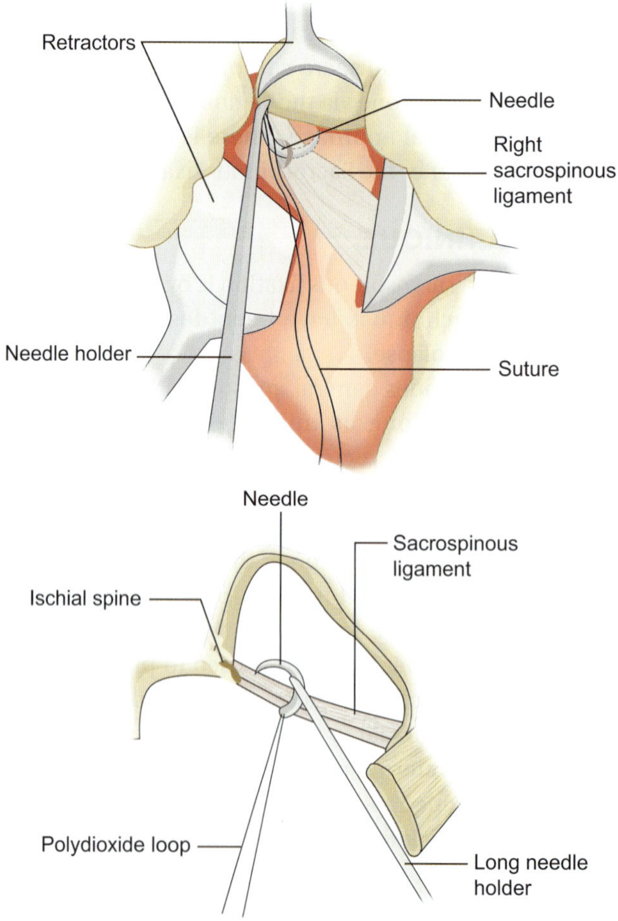

Fig. 4: Presentation of the procedure.

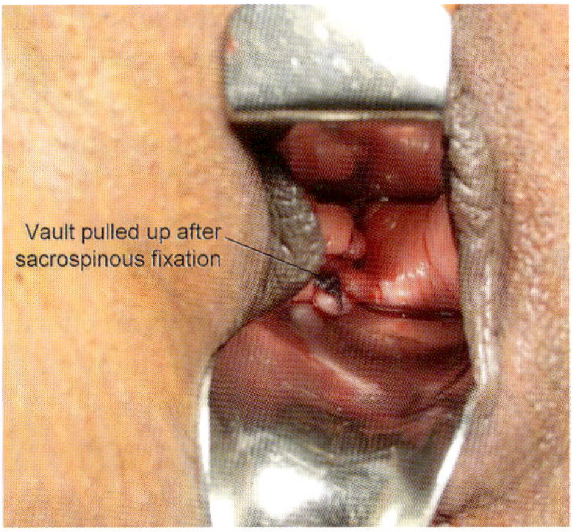

Fig. 5: The suspended vault after sacrospinous fixation.
Courtesy: Dr Rajshree Dayanand Katke

direct contact with the vaginal epithelium. Vault suspension is achieved as the healing process fuses the vaginal epithelium with the sacrospinous ligament. A course of broad-spectrum antibiotics can then be given post operatively.

Recently there has been a newer approach which uses a minimally invasive approach under visual guidance. This technique uses a suture catching device and a chipmunk tip endoscope to perform the fixation. The direct visualization of the ligament and suture place under the nanoscope guidance could be an advantage in terms of safety and better suture placement.

The complications that could arise as a result of Sacrospinous fixation are:

- Injury to the pudendal nerve
- Injury to the internal pudendal vessels
- Injury to the ureter
- Injury to the rectum

Other post operative complications could be:

- UTI
- Cuff cellulitis
- Ischiorectal abscess
- Cystocele
- Enterocele
- Shortening of the vaginal length which could leads to dyspareunia.

Beer and Kuhn reviewed the literature and found that the failure rates ranged from 3% to 37%. Further analysis showed that failure rates were higher in the anterior compartment and lower in the posterior and apical compartment. A meta-analysis showed that uterosacral ligament suspension is a highly effective procedure to restore the apical vaginal support. In a study by Nicholas, damage to the femoral and sciatic nerves were reported in 1.8%, gluteal pain, bladder pain, or unclassified pain in 0.8% and with the development of vaginal adhesions rectovaginal fistula in 0.5% of patients respectively.

CONCLUSION

Transvaginal sacrospinous colpopexy/fixation is an effective procedure and can be performed together with vaginal hysterectomy for prevention of huge prolapsed cases and in the treatment of vault prolapse.

ACKNOWLEDGMENT

The authors are grateful to authors/editors/publishers of all those articles, journals and books from where the literature for this article has been reviewed and discussed.

SUGGESTED READING

1. Beer M, Kuhn A. Surgical techniques for vault prolapse: a review of the literature. Eur J Obstetgynecolreprod Biol. 2005;119:14455.
2. Chene G, Cerruto E, Moret S, Nohuz E. The minimally invasive sacrospinous fixation under visual guidance: An anatomical study. Eur J Obstet Gynecol Reprod Biol. 2024;297:36-9.
3. Delancey OL. Vaginographic examination of the pelvic floor. Inturogynec J. 1994;5:19-24.
4. Gupta P. Transvaginal Sacrospinous Ligament Fixation for Pelvic Organ Prolapse Stage III and Stage IV Uterovaginal and Vault Prolapse. Iran J Med Sci. 2015;40(1):58-62.
5. Katke RD. (2016). Sacrospinous fixation: an efficient technique for prevention and treatment of vault prolapse. [online] Available from https://www.researchgate.net/publication/307974671 [Last accessed January, 2026].
6. Morley GW, Delancey JO. Sacrospinous ligament fixation for eversion of the vagina. Am J Obstet Gynecol. 1988;158:872-81.
7. Nichols DH, Randall CL. Vaginal surgery, 3rd edition. Baltimore: Williams Wilkins; 1989. pp. 339-48.
8. Persu C, Chapple CR, Cauni V, Gutue S, Geavlete P. Pelvic organ prolapse quantification system (pop-q)-a new era in pelvic prolapse staging. J Med Life. 2011;4:75-81.
9. Randall CL, Nichols DH. Surgical treatment of vaginal inversion. Obstet Gynecol. 1971;38:327-32.
10. Silva WA, Pauls RN, Segal JL, Rooney CM, Kleeman SD, Karram MM. Uterosacral ligament vault suspension: five-year outcomes. Obstet gynecol. 2006;108:255-63.

12 CHAPTER

Surgical Management of Pelvic Organs Prolapse

Nilakshi Phukan Kumar

INTRODUCTION

Pelvic organ prolapse (POP) is the descent of one or more of the anterior vaginal wall, posterior vaginal wall, the uterus, or the apex of the vagina (vaginal vault after hysterectomy). It affects up to 40–50% of parous women. Surgical correction remains the mainstay of management for symptomatic moderate-to-severe prolapse or when conservative therapies fail. Surgery aims to restore pelvic anatomy, improve functional outcomes, and reduce recurrence while maintaining sexual and urinary function. The choice of procedure depends on age, degree of prolapse, previous surgeries, sexual activity, and fertility desires. This review discusses commonly performed surgeries for POP, their techniques, indications, outcomes, advantages, and limitations based on current evidence.

NIH TERMINOLOGY WORKSHOP FOR RESEARCHERS IN FEMALE PELVIC FLOOR DISORDERS, 2001

POP was described:

- Anterior vaginal prolapse
- Apical or uterine prolapse
- Posterior vaginal prolapse

TYPES OF PROLAPSE

- Anterior—cystocele, urethrocystocele
- Apical—uterine prolapse, vaginal vault prolapse
- Posterior—enterocele, rectocele

SURGERY FOR POP

Reconstructive and Obliterative

Goals of pelvic reconstructive surgery

- Repair all the defects
- Restoration of normal anatomy
- Maintain normal vaginal function
- Improve symptoms related to POP

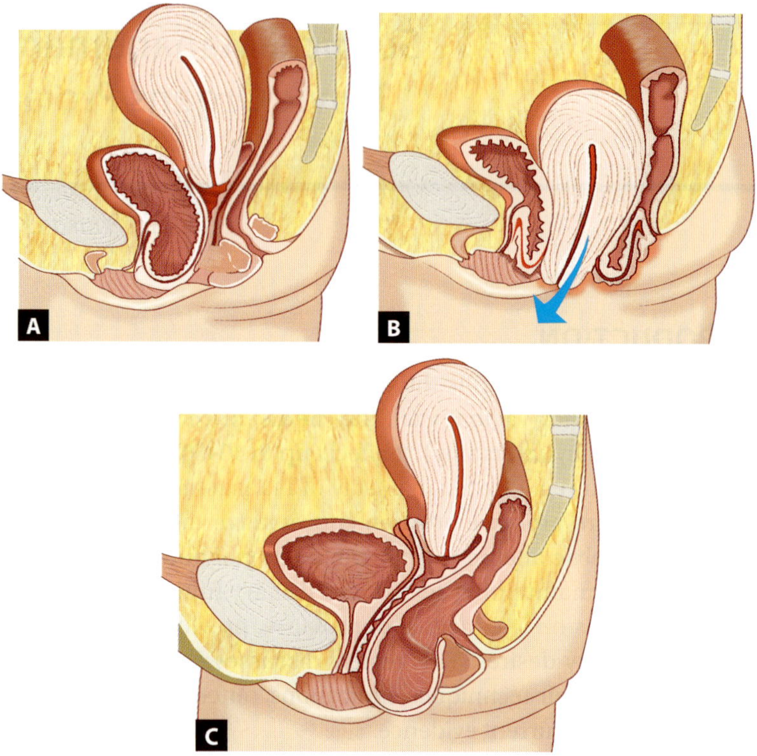

Figs. 1A to C: Diagram of types of Prolapse (A) Anterior, (B) Apical, (C) Posterior
Courtesy: From IUGA website: http://www.iugastore.com/en/pfd-anatomical-andsurgical-chart/98-pfd-anatomical-and-surgical-chart.html

- Improve Quality of Life
- Prevent recurrence

Route of pelvic reconstructive surgery

- Transvaginal
- Transabdominal
- Laparoscopy
  - Choice based on type and severity of POP, surgeon's training/ experience, patient's preference.

VAGINAL HYSTERECTOMY WITH PELVIC FLOOR REPAIR

Vaginal hysterectomy combined with anterior and posterior colporrhaphy is a widely performed surgery for uterine prolapse among women who have completed childbearing. McCall culdoplasty is often integrated to provide apical support and prevent future vault prolapse by approximating the uterosacral ligaments to the vaginal cuff.

Advantages

- Avoids an abdominal incision,
- Reduces postoperative pain,
- Offers excellent exposure to vaginal compartments
- High patient satisfaction.

LIMITATIONS

- Risk of recurrent apical prolapse if the apical suspension is inadequate.
- Over-tightening during posterior repair may cause dyspareunia.

UTERUS-SPARING SURGERIES (HYSTEROPEXY)

Uterine preservation has gained popularity, especially among younger women, those who desire future fertility, or women preferring to retain their uterus for cultural, sexual, or personal reasons. Evidence suggests that uterus-preserving procedures do not compromise outcomes when appropriately selected, and may offer faster recovery and improved sexual function.

Sacrospinous Hysteropexy (SSH)

In SSH, the cervix or uterus is suspended to the sacrospinous ligament via a vaginal approach. It is suitable for women with predominant uterine descent. Studies demonstrate that it provides comparable support to vagina while preserving the uterus. Risks include buttock pain, pudendal nerve irritation, and altered vaginal axis.

Uterosacral Ligament Hysteropexy

This technique utilizes native uterosacral ligaments to suspend the uterus. Laparoscopic or vaginal approaches may be used. It avoids mesh use and maintains anatomical vaginal axis. However, ureteric injury is a recognized complication due to proximity of the ureter to the uterosacral ligaments.

Laparoscopic or Abdominal Sacrohysteropexy

This is a mesh-based procedure involving attachment of the uterus to the sacral promontory using a synthetic mesh. This approach achieves excellent apical support, with long-term success rates exceeding 90% in several series. It also preserves vaginal length and function. However, mesh-related complications (1–10%), need for advanced surgical skills, and longer operative time are potential disadvantages.

ANTERIOR COLPORRHAPHY

Anterior colporrhaphy is performed to repair cystocele by reinforcing the pubocervical fascia. It is simple, quick, and associated with minimal morbidity. Despite its widespread use, recurrence rates are relatively high (up to 30–40% in

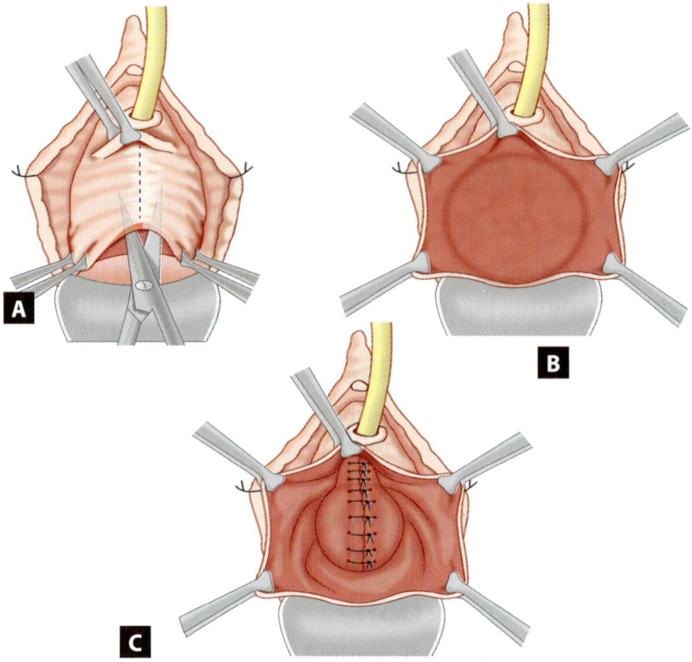

Figs. 2A to C: Anterior colporrhaphy.
Courtesy: Adapted from Uptodate:https://www.uptodate.com/contents/image?imageKey=OBGYN%2F51734&topicKey=OBGYN%2F15268&source=outline_link&search=Partial%20colpocleisis%20&selectedTitle=1~150

some long-term studies). Synthetic mesh augmentation theoretically provides more durable support, but due to concerns over mesh erosion, dyspareunia, and regulatory restrictions, mesh is now avoided in primary anterior repairs in many countries. The procedure remains useful for mild to moderate cystocele but may require adjunct apical suspension in large defects.

POSTERIOR COLPORRHAPHY

Posterior colporrhaphy is performed for posterior compartment prolapse It is typically performed via the vaginal route with low complication rates. However, over-correction may result in dyspareunia. Recurrence is lower than in anterior repairs, partly due to stronger posterior fascial support.

Posterior Compartment Prolapse (Rectocele/Enterocele)

- Native Tissue Repairs
  - Posterior Colporrhaphy
    - Plication of rectovaginal fascia.
  - Site-specific Repair
    - Targeted re-approximation of fascia defects.

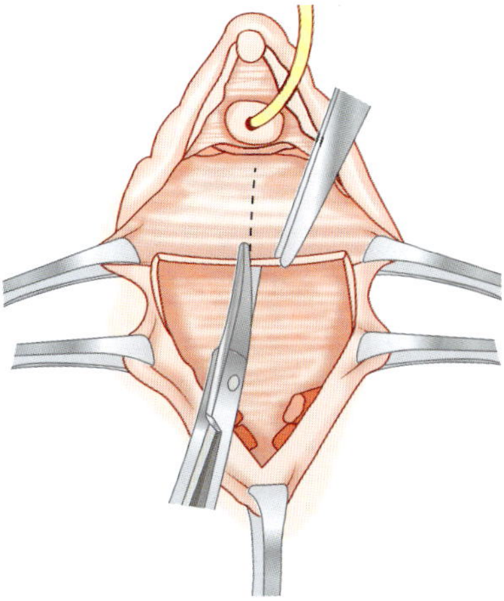

Fig. 3: Posterior colporrhaphy.

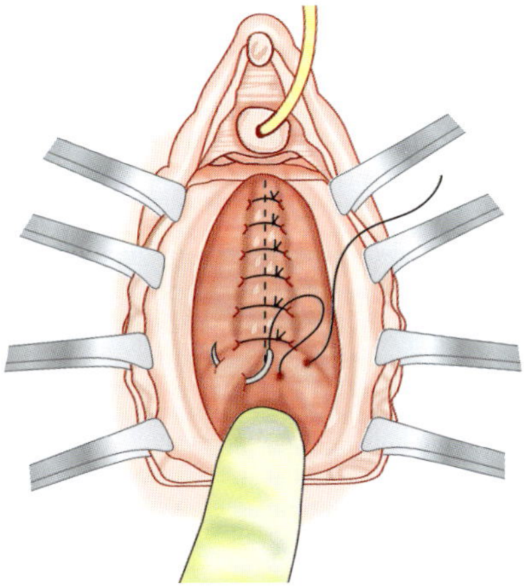

Fig. 4: Posterior colporrhaphy.

Courtesy: Adapted from Uptodate:https://www.uptodate.com/contents/image?imageKey=OBGYN%2F51734&topicKey=OBGYN%2F15268&source=outline_link&search=Partial%20colpocleisis%20&selectedTitle=1~150

  - Perineorrhaphy
    - Reconstruction of the perineal body.
- Enterocele Repairs
  - McCall culdoplasty (after vaginal hysterectomy)
  - Moschcowitz procedure (abdominal purse-string of cul-de-sac)
  - Laparoscopic uterosacral ligament suspension

SACROCOLPOPEXY/SACROHYSTEROPEXY

Sacrocolpopexy is widely regarded as the gold standard for apical prolapse, especially in sexually active women or those requiring long-term durable correction. It involves attaching the vaginal vault (post-hysterectomy) or uterus (hysteropexy) to the sacral promontory using polypropylene mesh. The procedure can be performed via open abdominal, laparoscopic, or robotic routes.

Advantages

- Superior long-term success rates (>90%)
- Maintains vaginal length, axis, and sexual function
- Lower recurrence of apical and multi-compartment defects
- Preferred in recurrent prolapse or young women needing durability

Disadvantages

- Mesh-related complications including erosion, infection, or pain
- Risk of presacral hemorrhage
- Longer operative time and need for advanced laparoscopic skills.

Current evidence, including the CARE, OPUS, and PROPEL trials, supports sacrocolpopexy as the most durable option for vault prolapse, with mesh erosion rates of around 3–10% depending on material and technique.

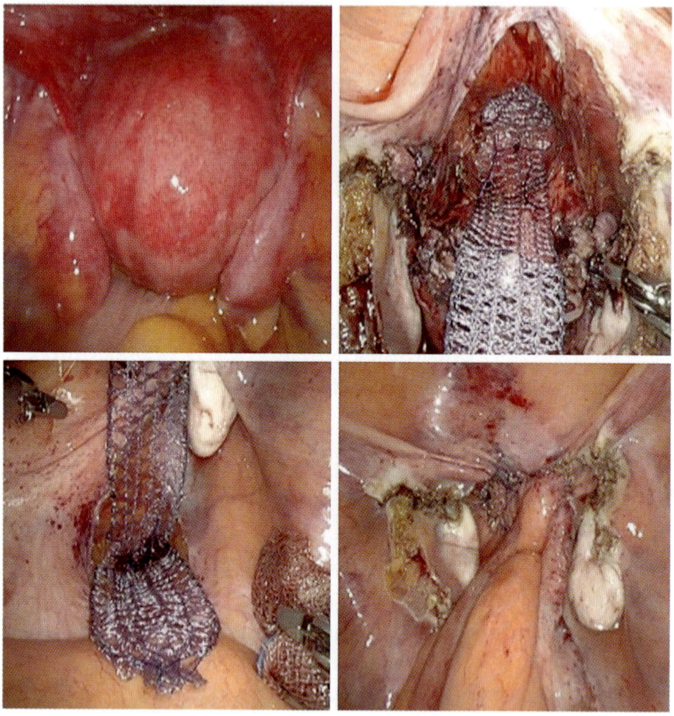

Fig. 5: Laparoscopic sacrocolpopexy.

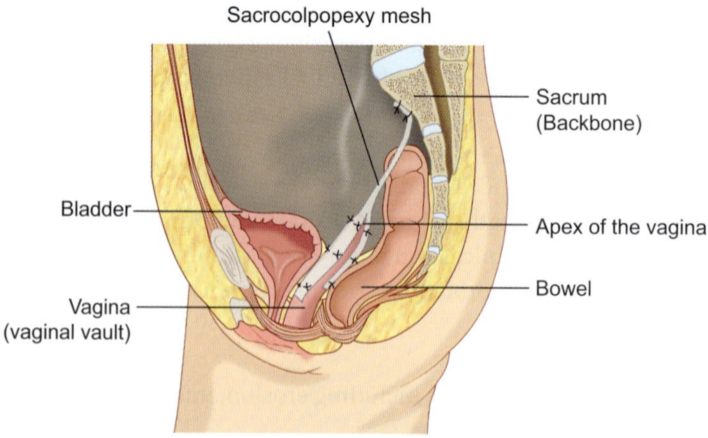

Fig. 6: Sacrocolpopexy.

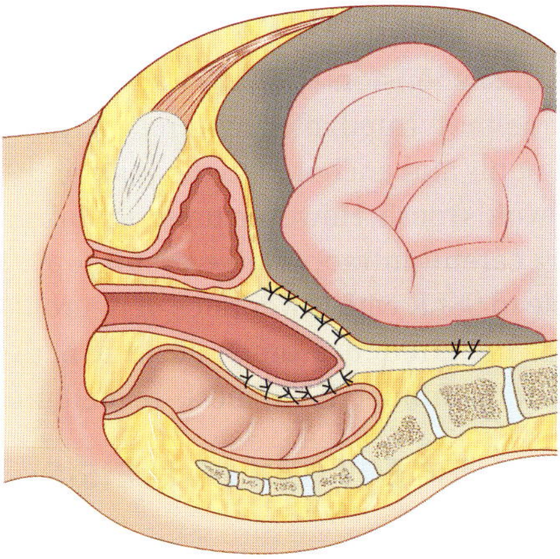

Fig. 7: Sacrocolpexy.
Courtesy: Adapted from Uptodate:https://www.uptodate.com/contents/image?imageKey=OBGYN%2F51734&topicKey=OBGYN%2F15268&source=outline_link&search=Partial%20colpocleisis%20&selectedTitle=1~150

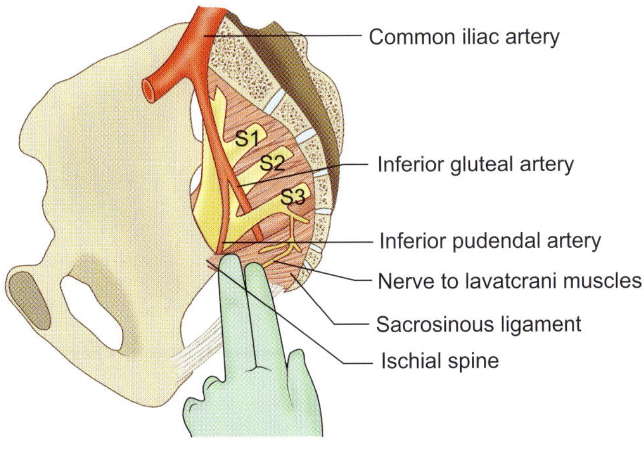

Fig. 8: Anatomy of sacrospinous ligament.
Courtesy: https://www.jsafog.com/abstractArticleContentBrowse/JSAFOG/21658/JPJ

Sacrospinous Ligament Fixation (SSLF)

Sacrospinous ligament fixation (SSLF) is a native tissue repair performed via the vaginal route and is commonly used for post-hysterectomy vaginal vault prolapse. The apex of the vagina is attached to the sacrospinous ligament, usually unilaterally. The procedure avoids mesh use and abdominal entry, making it attractive for older women or those with multiple comorbidities. Success rates range between 75–90%.

Limitations include alteration of vaginal axis, buttock pain, and possible pudendal nerve injury. Compared to sacrocolpopexy, SSLF may have a higher risk of anterior compartment recurrence due to posterior tethering of the apex.

UTEROSACRAL LIGAMENT SUSPENSION

Uterosacral ligament suspension (USLS) is a native-tissue vaginal apical suspension technique performed after hysterectomy. Sutures are placed in the uterosacral ligaments and anchored to the vaginal cuff. It provides strong apical support and avoids mesh. However, ureteric kinking or obstruction can occur, necessitating careful intraoperative cystoscopy. Long-term success rates are comparable to SSLF, with lower rates of neuropathic pain.

This procedure is preferred for women desiring native tissue repair with high apical support and minimal risk of mesh-related problems.

OBLITERATIVE SURGERY (COLPOCLEISIS)

Colpocleisis is an obliterative procedure suitable for elderly women who are not sexually active and have no desire for future vaginal intercourse. It involves partial or complete closure of the vaginal canal, typically through a Le Fort procedure. It has very high success rates (~95%), minimal complications, and is particularly useful in frail patients. However, it precludes vaginal cervical or uterine assessment, so preoperative evaluation for uterine pathology is essential.

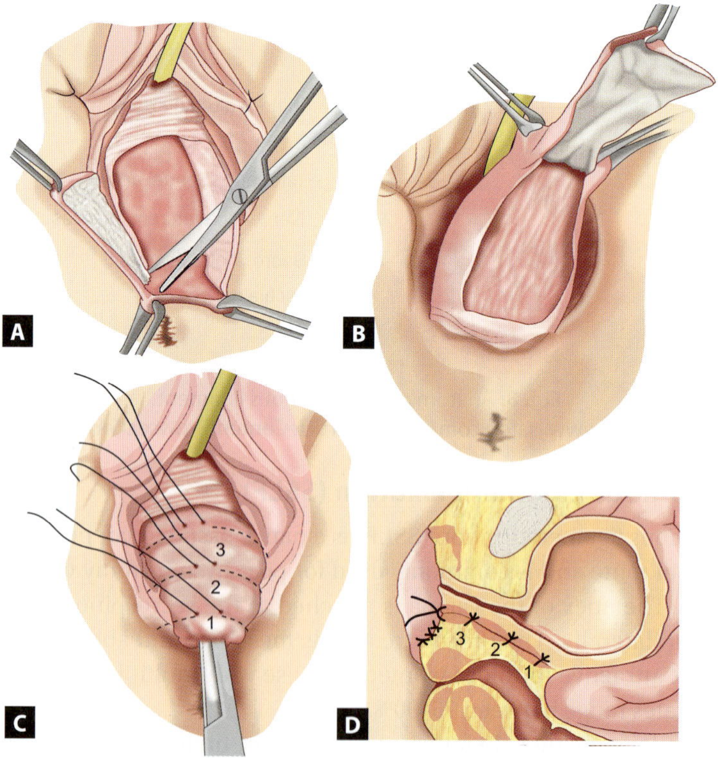

Figs. 9A to D: Le Fort colpocleisis.
Courtesy: https://obgynkey.com/obliterative-procedures-for-pelvic-organ-prolapse-2

CHOOSING THE RIGHT PROCEDURE

The optimal surgery is individualized based on the patient's age, sexual and reproductive requirements, prolapse stage, compartment involvement, and comorbidities. General principles include:

- *Young women or those desiring fertility:* Uterus-preserving procedures (sacrohysteropexy preferred for durability)
- *Severe apical prolapse:* Sacrocolpopexy offers best long-term outcomes
- *Mild to moderate cystocele/rectocele:* Native tissue repairs
- *Post-hysterectomy vault prolapse:* SSLF or USLS
- *Elderly, not sexually active:* Colpocleisis
- *Recurrent prolapse:* Sacrocolpopexy or mesh-based hysteropexy.

CONCLUSION

Surgical management of pelvic organ prolapse encompasses a range of procedures targeting different pelvic compartments and addressing individual patient needs. Although vaginal hysterectomy with pelvic floor repair remains a traditional and effective approach, uterus-sparing surgeries have gained acceptance due to comparable outcomes and better patient satisfaction. Sacrocolpopexy continues to be the gold standard for apical prolapse due to its superior long-term success rates, while native-tissue repairs such as SSLF and USLS offer effective alternatives without the risks associated with mesh. Obliterative procedures remain important for selected elderly women. Comprehensive evaluation, individualized planning, and evidence-based surgical selection are key to optimizing outcomes and reducing recurrence.

SUGGESTED READING

1. ACOG Practice Bulletin No. 214: Pelvic Organ Prolapse. American College of Obstetricians and Gynecologists, 2019.
2. Barber MD. Operations and Pelvic Muscle Training in the Management of Apical Support Loss (OPTIMAL) trial. JAMA. 2014;311(10):1023-34.
3. Bump RC, Norton PA. Epidemiology and natural history of pelvic floor dysfunction. Obstet Gynecol Clin North Am. 1998;25:723-46.
4. FDA Safety Communication: Vaginal mesh for POP repair. USA: US Food and Drug Administration; 2019.
5. Food and Drug Administration. Urogynecologic surgical mesh: update on the safety and effectiveness of transvaginal placement for pelvic organ prolapse. USA: Food and Drug Administration; 2011.
6. Haylen BT, de Ridder D, Freeman RM, Swift SE, Berghmans B, Lee J, et al. International Urogynecological Association; International Continence Society. An International Urogynecological Association (IUGA)/International Continence Society (ICS) joint report on the terminology for female pelvic floor dysfunction. Neurourol Urodyn. 2010;29:4–20.

7. Iglesia CB, Smithling KR. Pelvic Organ Prolapse. Am Fam Physician. 2017; 96:179-85.
8. LeFort. De la gynaptysie. Presse Med Belge. 187
9. Maher C, et al. Surgical management of pelvic organ prolapse. Int Urogynecol J. 2013;24:1781-92.
10. Meyer I, McGwin G, Swain TA, Alvarez MD, Ellington DR, Richter HE. Synthetic graft augmentation in vaginal prolapse surgery: long-term objective and subjective outcomes. J Minim Invasive Gynecol. 2016;23:614-21.
11. NICE. (2019). Urinary incontinence and pelvic organ prolapse in women: management. NICE guideline NG123. [online] Available from https://www.nice.org.uk/guidance/ng123 [Last accessed January, 2026]
12. Nygaard I, Brubaker L, Zyczynski HM, Cundiff G, Richter H, Gantz M, et al. Long-term outcomes following abdominal sacrocolpopexy. JAMA. 2013; 309(19):2016-24.
13. Weber AM, Walters MD. Review of anatomy and techniques of surgical repair. Obstet Gynecol. 1997;89:311-8.

13 CHAPTER

Medical Management of Pelvic Organ Prolapse

Ashok Kumar Todani

INTRODUCTION

Something coming down per vagina is a frequent complain by parous ladies, and by nulliparous sometimes. Since it is a phenomenon of pelvic viscera, particularly reproductive organs, POP or pelvic organ prolapse is commonly used term for it. It is a rampant prevalent condition in the female population. It jeopardizes confidence and thus quality of life is lowered due to reduced capability. Many publications and data point towards conflicting causes and their effect.

Before considering treatment options, one has to consider in depth different conceptual types of female reproductive organ anatomy, like structural, positional, functional, pathological and surgical anatomy. All these parameters are different in nulliparous and multiparous women influenced by their socio-economic status. We have to search for obstetric events or other risk factors that could play a central role in the prevention of ultimate prolapse.

Most pelvic viscera are supported and positioned jointly by pelvic fasciae and muscles. So their importance should always be estimated with due attention. With rise in demand for uterine preservation, surgical trends are currently changing. Literature is available linking libido with presence of uterus, cervix in particular.

Since prolapse is a matter of position [downward displacement from normal position], positional anatomy of uterus and vagina needs considerable attention. Pathological anatomy is structural anatomy in its altered state. Implied in this statement is also the altered functional anatomy that runs parallel with it. Root cause of prolapse is loss of support to the uterus, urinary bladder and bowel. This leads to their descent along an axis from their normal anatomical situs towards or through the vaginal introitus.

Using PV examination as a criteria, the incidence of POP varies between 30–40 percent. Studies and their data suggest 6 to 8% of women complain of a bulging mass sensation per vaginum. POP leads to depressed personality of affected lady as far as psychological, physical, emotional and social wellbeing is concerned. This leads to huge resource depletion due to 'health loss.'

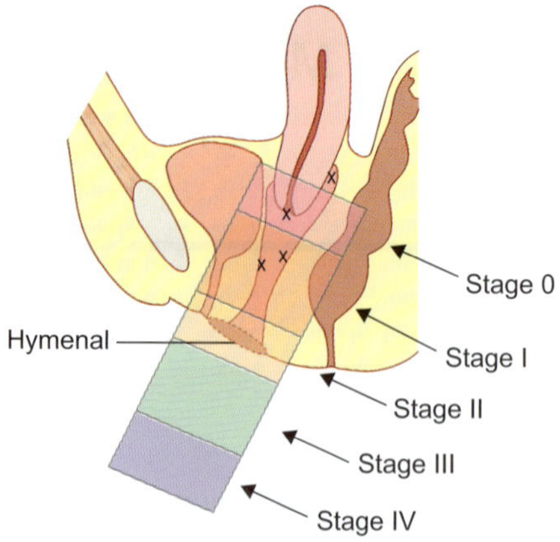

Fig. 1: Causes and progress of prolapse.

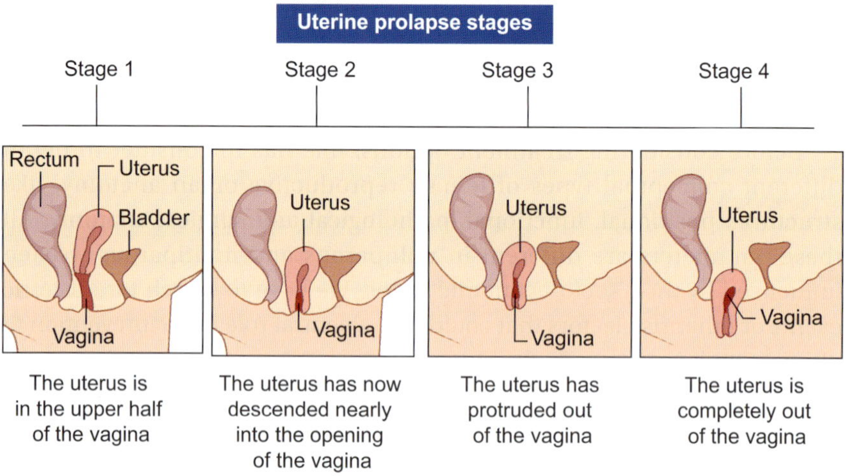

Fig. 2: Degrees of prolapse.

Modern health care system is putting more emphasis on prevention rather than cure. There are examples of preventive aspects in community medicine in preventing pelvic floor dysfunction or weakness which are leading to prolapse, but they are in infantry stage. Specially in elderly and grand multipara going in labor at an older age, demand for conservative management and preservation of uterus increases in an ageing population. We should briefly take into account different situations and discuss them regarding prevention measures, and conservative options in cases of pelvic organ prolapse.

Different and prevalent disposing risk factors inducing and promoting POP are:

- Occupational hazards, e.g., heavy weight lifting and straining downwards
- *Lifestyle modification factors:* Obesity, Smoking, COPD, strenuous exercise etc.

- *Altered Bowel function:* Chronic constipation and habitual defecatory straining, consumption of diet deficient in roughage.
- Obstetric factors like high parity, vaginal delivery, instrumental vaginal delivery
- Age factor particularly postmenopausal status
- Pelvic surgery particularly Hysterectomy, Pelvic organ prolapse surgery, colposuspension, rectopexy, and many more.
- Different Congenital connective tissue disorders like Ehlers-Danlos/ Benign joint hypermobility syndrome, Marfan syndrome, and prevalent family history

The medical management of pelvic organ prolapse (POP) primarily involves nonsurgical options such as pelvic muscle exercises, pessaries, and lifestyle modifications to alleviate symptoms and improve quality of life.

NONSURGICAL MANAGEMENT OPTIONS

Pelvic Muscle Exercises

Kegel Exercises: These exercises strengthen the pelvic floor muscles, which can help support the pelvic organs and may alleviate some symptoms associated with prolapse. While they do not reverse the prolapse, they can improve muscle tone and reduce urinary incontinence.

Pessaries

Vaginal Support Devices: Pessaries are silicone devices inserted into the vagina to support the pelvic organs and alleviate symptoms. They are a safe, cost-effective, and minimally invasive option for managing POP. Pessaries can be used as a first-line treatment, especially for women who prefer to avoid surgery.

Follow-up care on a regular basis with utmost sincerity is a must to ensure proper fitting and absence of any complications like vaginal irritation, ulceration etc..

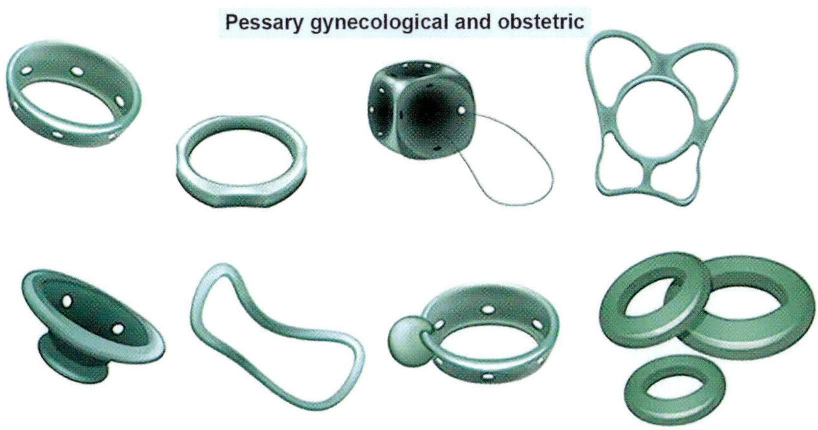

Fig. 3: Different types of pessaries used.

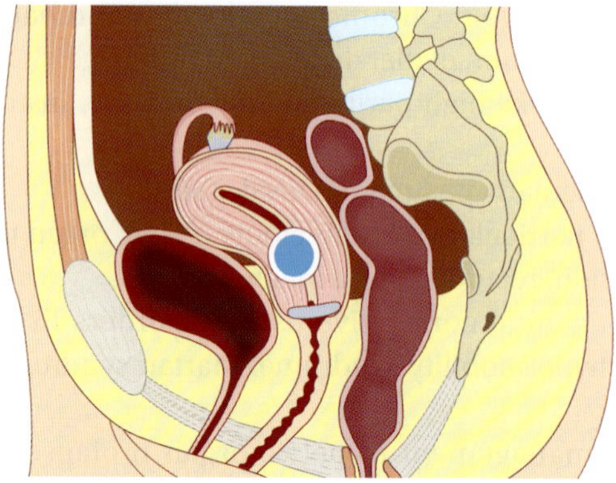

Fig. 4: Vaginal pessary applied in place.

Topical Estrogen

For women experiencing atrophic vaginitis or signs of hypoestrogenism, the application of topical estrogen may be beneficial. This can improve vaginal tissue health and enhance the effectiveness of pessary use.

Urogenital atrophy is frequently seen in conjunction with prolapse. As revealed by certain studies, estrogens alone or in conjunction with other measures, may prevent or retard the development of such atrophic changes by improving the strength of weakened supporting ligaments, muscles and vaginal mucosa. However, there is varying evidence to support or endorse this hypothesis. If we consider results from studies regarding lower urinary tract symptoms and hormone replacement therapy, local estrogen treatments appear more promising compared to systemic administration. We are in dire need for rigorous many more randomized controlled trials, with long-term follow-up, to assess estrogen preparations for the prevention of pelvic organ prolapse.

"Cheung et al" found that prolapse symptoms and quality of life improved in women with symptomatic stage I to stage III POP using a vaginal medicated pessary in addition to pelvic floor exercises.

LIFESTYLE MODIFICATIONS

Weight Management: Maintaining a healthy weight can reduce pressure on the pelvic floor.

Heavy weight lifting will increase intra-abdominal pressure thereby promoting prolapse and exaggerating symptoms.

So, reducing such activities will definitely help and manage symptomatology.

One should eliminate or modify other risk factors which can help us lower the risk of POP. Reducing straining and intra-abdominal pressure rise can help prevent the development of prolapse. The widely accepted practice of treatment of bowel dysfunction/chronic constipation has not been tested as systematic intervention to prevent pelvic organ prolapse. Weight loss using high roughage diet is helpful. Bariatric surgery leading to weight reduction has been suggested as a good preventive measure. Few published cohort studies with short-term follow-up have shown that weight reduction is associated with subjective improvement in prolapse symptoms but no objective change was seen in examination using the pelvic organ prolapse quantification (POP-Q) system.

Smoking quitting improves respiratory system compliance improving oxygen status

NONSURGICAL TREATMENT

Nonsurgical management comprises of physical interventions to improve the function and support of the pelvic floor muscles (via pelvic floor muscle training) and mechanical interventions (insertion of vaginal pessaries) to support the prolapse. They are often offered for lower grades of prolapse and to women unwilling or unfit to undergo surgery.

Pessaries

Since days of yore, a wide variety of different items are being used to manage and treat urogenital prolapse. In trade, many types of medicated and non-medicated vaginal pessaries are available. Pessaries are mainly of two types: supporting and space-occupying means.

A recent Cochrane review has highlighted the lack of robust evidence regarding the effectiveness of vaginal pessaries.

But 77% of the members of the American Urogynecologic Society use pessaries as first-line therapy.

As there is no evidence to support the use of a specific type, choice is based on experience and trial and error. With successful insertion of pessary, there is significant improvement in prolapse symptoms, and in bladder, bowel and sexual function.

Vaginal pessaries are manufactured from medical-grade silicone and are expected to be safe, cost-effective, and minimally invasive options for treating patients with pelvic organ prolapse. Data suggest that pessary use has few contraindications relatively: lack of patient's ability to comply with follow-up and instructions (e.g., dementia), vaginal fistulas, uterovaginal erosions, and undiagnosed uterovaginal bleeding. Application of topical estrogen prior to pessary use is an important adjunct, particularly if signs of hypo-estrogenism (atrophic vaginitis) exist. Once the pessary is in place, continued vaginal estrogen cream application (i.e., 1–2 times per week) or application of a vaginal estrogen ring once every 3 months is indicated, unless estrogen is contraindicated (like estrogen-dependent breast tumor or other alike situations). Vaginal erosions and discharge are indications for temporary pessary removal and treatment with topical estrogen.

Pelvic Floor Muscle Training

Kegel exercises are beneficial for women to strengthen pelvic floor muscles. Here's how to perform them:
Correct and suitable muscle needs to be identified for therapy by stopping urination midway. These muscles need attention for treatment.

Performing Kegels

The patient has to first empty urinary bladder and find the right muscle by pretending to stop urinary flow. Then tighten and hold these muscles for 3–5 seconds, followed by 3–5 seconds rest. Repeat this 10 times per set, and aim for three sets per day.

One has to locate correct Pelvic Floor Muscles in question so that doing Kegel exercises will benefit them. One should imagine that she is urinating. She should tighten the muscles she would use to stop the stream of urine. Those are her pelvic floor muscles needed to be exercised. She should not stop urine stream midway to avoid risk for a UTI. Tightening the muscles she would use to hold back a bowel movement or keep herself away from passing gas. Placing the tip of a clean finger into her vagina and tightening her pelvic floor muscles around her finger, she should feel her vagina tighten and her pelvic floor move upward.

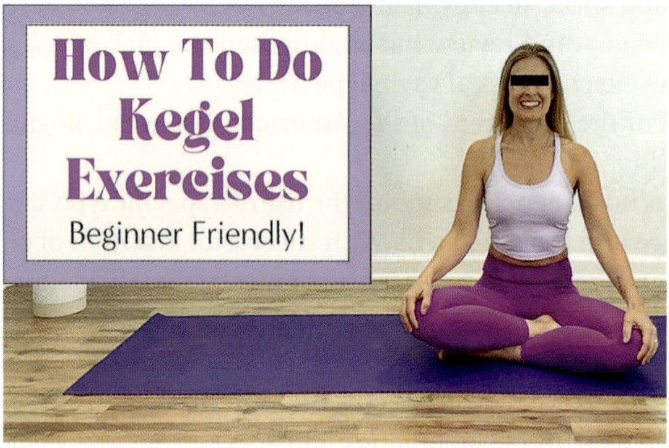

Fig. 5: Doing Kegel exercise.

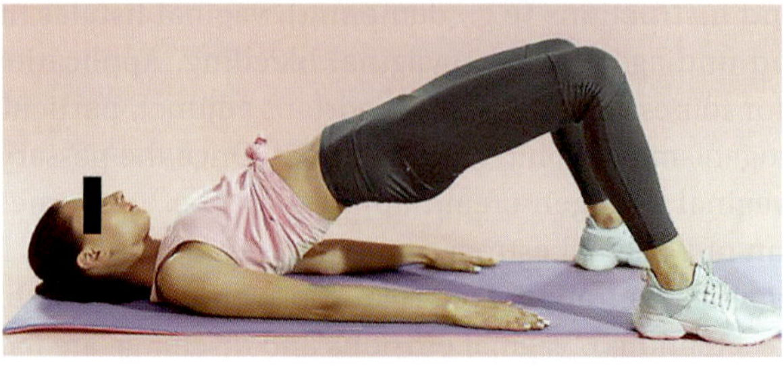

Fig. 6: Posture during Kegel exercise.

Benefits

This will help her prevent urinary incontinence and pelvic floor problems. It can improve her sexual health and satisfaction.

Tips

She should avoid tightening her abdomen, thighs, or buttocks during the exercises. It should be a daily routine.

WHAT IS THE EMSELLA CHAIR?

The Emsella Chair is an FDA-approved, non-invasive treatment that uses high-intensity focused electromagnetic (HIFEM) energy to target and stimulate the pelvic floor muscles.

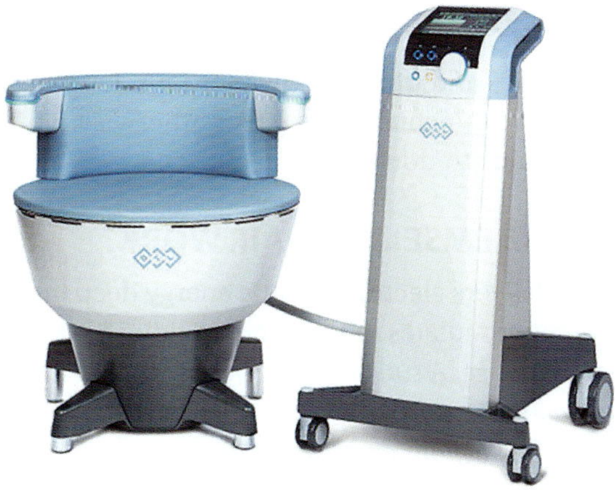

Fig. 7: Emsella chair.

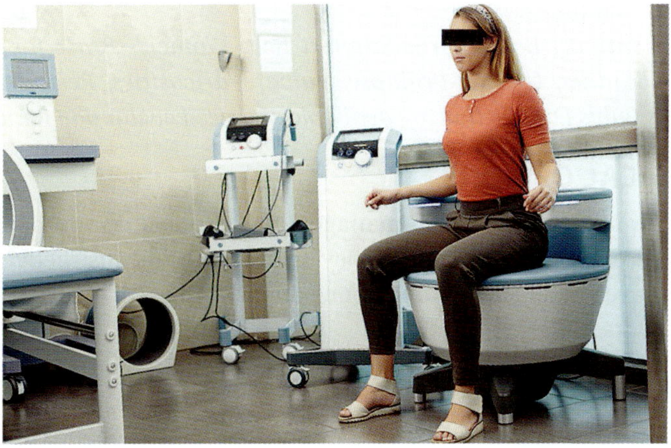

Fig. 8: Patient sitting comfortably for treatment.

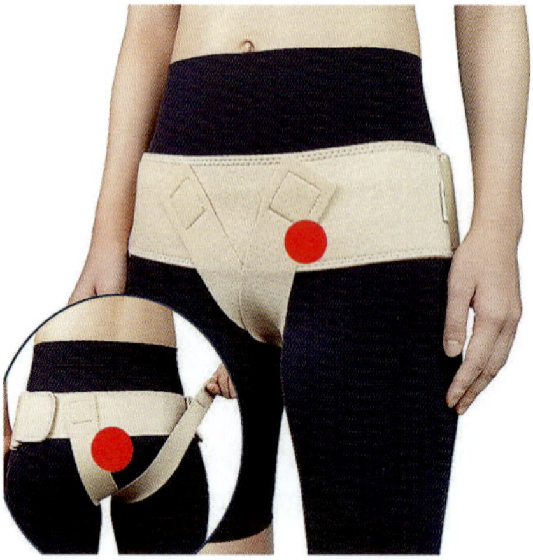

Fig. 9: Pelvic support belt for prolapse.

The chair stimulates and trains pelvic floor muscles making them strong and tight. It is difficult to achieve this effect otherwise. This effort doesn't involve any drug administration as well.

HOW DOES THE EMSELLA CHAIR WORK?

The Emsella Chair delivers electromagnetic energy deep into the pelvic floor muscles. This energy stimulates muscle contractions far more powerful than the average Kegel exercise. *A single session in the Emsella Chair can stimulate over 11,000 contractions, more than any woman could achieve on her own through traditional pelvic floor exercises.*

These intense contractions cause the muscles to strengthen over time, improving bladder control, enhancing sexual health, and reducing the risk of prolapse. Think of it like a workout for your pelvic muscles but without any of the sweat or strain.

Pelvic Support Belt, Uterus Support Belt, Women's Brace for Treating Dropped Bladder, Uterine Prolapse, Vulvar Varicosities, Postpartum and Symphysis Pubis Dysfunction are available and need evaluation for use.

SURGICAL OPTIONS

In event of failure of medical management, surgical option needs to be considered. Surgical interventions may be in form of reconstructive surgery, or obliterative surgery depending upon patient's preference. Sexual activities need be addressed.

CONCLUSION

The conservative management of pelvic organ prolapse depends upon needs and preference of patient guided by personal needs. Nonsurgical options like pelvic muscle exercise and pelvic floor rejuvenation, pessary (aided by local estrogen supplementation) are useful first line management.

One should advocate treatment that can significantly improve quality of life of patient suffering from POP. Regular follow up and life style modifications are crucial components foe effective management.

ACKNOWLEDGMENT

I am thankful and obliged to Dr Rishi Todani for his support to typeset this article.

SUGGESTED READING

1. Abdool Z, Thakar R, Sultan AH, Oliver RS. Prospective evaluation of outcome of vaginal pessaries versus surgery in women with symptomatic pelvic organ prolapse. Int Urogynecol J. 2011;22:273-8.
2. Braekken IH, Majida M, Engh ME, Bø K. Can pelvic floor muscle training reverse pelvic organ prolapse and reduce prolapse symptoms? An assessor-blinded, randomized, controlled trial. Am J Obstet Gynecol. 2010;203:170.e1-7.
3. Bugge C, Adams EJ, Gopinath D, Reid F. Pessaries (mechanical devices) for pelvic organ prolapse in women. Cochrane Database Syst Rev. 2013;2:CD004010.
4. Cody JD, Jacobs ML, Richardson K, Moehrer B, Hextall A. Oestrogen therapy for urinary incontinence in post-menopausal women. Cochrane Database Syst Rev. 2012;10:CD001405.
5. Cuicchi D, Lombardi R, Cariani S, Leuratti L, Lecce F, Cola B. Clinical and instrumental evaluation of pelvic floor disorders before and after bariatric surgery in obese women. Surg Obes Relat Dis. 2013;9:69-75.
6. Cundiff GW, Weidner AC, Visco AG, Bump RC, Addison WA. A survey of pessary use by members of the American urogynecologic society. Obstet Gynecol. 2000;95:931-5.
7. Digesu GA, Khullar V, Cardozo L, Robinson D, Salvatore S. P-QOL: a validated questionnaire to assess the symptoms and quality of life of women with urogenital prolapse. Int Urogynecol J Pelvic Floor Dysfunct. 2005;16: 176-81.
8. Glazener C, Elders A, Macarthur C, Lancashire RJ, Herbison P, Hagen S, et al. Childbirth and prolapse: long-term associations with the symptoms and objective measurement of pelvic organ prolapse. BJOG. 2013;120:16-8.
9. Gozukara YM, Akalan G, Tok EC, Aytan H, Ertunc D. The improvement in pelvic floor symptoms with weight loss in obese women does not correlate with the changes in pelvic anatomy. Int Urogynecol J. 2014;25:1219-25.
10. Hagen S, Stark D, Glazener C, Dickson S, Barry S, Elders A, et al. Individualised pelvic floor muscle training in women with pelvic organ prolapse (POPPY): a multicentre randomised controlled trial. Lancet. 2014;383:796-806.
11. Hendrix SL, Clark A, Nygaard I, Aragaki A, Barnabei V, McTiernan A. Pelvic organ prolapse in the Women's Health Initiative: gravity and gravidity. Am J Obstet Gynecol. 2002;186:1160-6.
12. Lawrence JM, Lukacz ES, Nager CW, Hsu JY, Luber KM. Prevalence and co-occurrence of pelvic floor disorders in community-dwelling women. Obstet Gynecol. 2008;111:678-85.

13. McClurg D, Hilton P, Dolan L, Monga A, Hagen S, Frawley H, et al. Pelvic floor muscle training as an adjunct to prolapse surgery: a randomised feasibility study. Int Urogynecol J. 2014;25:883-91.
14. Samuelsson EC, Victor FT, Tibblin G, Svärdsudd KF. Signs of genital prolapse in a Swedish population of women 20 to 59 years of age and possible related factors. Am J Obstet Gynecol. 1999;180:299-305.
15. Tegerstedt G, Maehle-Schmidt M, Nyrén O, Hammarström M. Prevalence of symptomatic pelvic organ prolapse in a Swedish population. Int Urogynecol J Pelvic Floor Dysfunct. 2005;16:497-503.
16. Ward RM, Velez Edwards Digna R, Edwards T, Giri A, Jerome RN, Wu JM. Genetic epidemiology of pelvic organ prolapse: a systematic revision. Am J Obstet Gynecol. 2014;S0002-9378:00344-5.
17. Wilson D, Dornan J, Milsom I, Freeman R. UR-CHOICE: can we provide mothers-to-be with information about the risk of future pelvic floor dysfunction? Int Urogynecol J. 2014;25(11):1449-52.

14 CHAPTER

Laparoscopic Cerclage

Ajay Aggarwal, Aarti Chitkara

INTRODUCTION

Cervical insufficiency represents a significant cause of spontaneous preterm birth, affecting approximately 1% of all pregnancies and accounting for nearly 8% of recurrent pregnancy losses. It is classically defined as a painless, progressive dilation of the cervix in the absence of uterine contractions, which culminates in recurrent mid-trimester pregnancy losses in women who otherwise have normal pregnancies. Cervical cerclage, a procedure in which a supporting suture is placed around the cervix, has long been recognized as an effective intervention to prolong pregnancy and reduce the incidence of preterm birth, neonatal morbidity, and mortality.

When transvaginal cerclage is not feasible or has previously failed, a transabdominal approach may be used. Evidence demonstrates that abdominal cerclage is highly effective at decreasing fetal loss and improving gestational outcomes in appropriately selected patients. It can be performed either before pregnancy (interval cerclage) or during early gestation. With modern minimally invasive surgery, *laparoscopic transabdominal cerclage (TAC)* has become the preferred technique due to reduced postoperative pain, quicker recovery, and lower operative morbidity compared with open laparotomy.

INDICATIONS FOR CERCLAGE

History-indicated Cerclage

A history-indicated cerclage is recommended for patients with a strong obstetric history suggestive of cervical insufficiency. This includes women with *three or more prior second-trimester losses* (beyond 16 weeks) or extremely preterm births attributed to cervical dilation rather than labor. ACOG also allows consideration of cerclage after *one unexplained mid-trimester loss,* underscoring individualized clinical judgment.

Previous Cerclage

Women with a prior cerclage require individualized assessment rather than an automatic repeat procedure. However, ACOG guidelines support offering a repeat cerclage in patients with a confirmed history of cervical insufficiency who have previously undergone the procedure.

Ultrasound-indicated Cerclage

Cerclage may be considered in ongoing singleton pregnancies when transvaginal ultrasound reveals *cervical shortening between 10 and 25 mm*, especially in the presence of prior preterm birth or other risk factors.

Physical Examination (Rescue) Cerclage

If a patient presents with *painless cervical dilation* on examination, rescue cerclage is recommended, provided membranes are intact and no contraindications exist.

INDICATIONS FOR TRANSABDOMINAL CERCLAGE

Transabdominal cerclage is more invasive than the transvaginal approach, particularly when performed via laparotomy. Therefore, *laparoscopic TAC* is generally preferred over laparotomy, as it offers the advantages of minimally invasive surgery.

We select patients for laparoscopic TAC based on the following criteria:

Inability to Perform Transvaginal Cerclage

This includes anatomical or pathological conditions such as:

- Severely shortened or absent cervix
- Cervical amputation
- Significant cervical scarring
- Congenital or acquired cervical defects

These conditions may make transvaginal suture placement technically impossible or unsafe.

Failed Transvaginal Cerclage

Laparoscopic TAC is appropriate when a *history-indicated or ultrasound-indicated vaginal cerclage has failed* in a previous pregnancy. Failure of an emergent (rescue) cerclage alone is not considered an indication.

Why is TAC more Effective

The abdominal approach provides several advantages:

- *Placement at the level of the internal os*, which is the anatomically optimal location.
- *Minimal risk of suture migration* as the uterus expands.
- *Reduced infection risk*, since no foreign body is placed in the vagina.

Laparoscopic versus Open Abdominal Cerclage

When performed by an experienced laparoscopic surgeon, the laparoscopic technique is not only comparable in efficacy to open TAC but is often superior, offering reduced blood loss, faster recovery, and fewer postoperative complications. Published series report high success rates for laparoscopic TAC with excellent pregnancy outcomes.

CONTRAINDICATIONS TO TAC

Contraindications align closely with those used for transvaginal cerclage and include:

- Fetal anomalies incompatible with life
- Intrauterine infection or chorioamnionitis
- Active uterine bleeding
- Active preterm labor
- Preterm prelabor rupture of membranes (PPROM)
- Fetal demise

Prolapsed membranes through the external os represent a relative contraindication due to an >50% risk of iatrogenic membrane rupture during manipulation.

TIMING OF TAC

Interval or Preconception Cerclage

Placing TAC before pregnancy offers several benefits:

- No risk to an existing pregnancy
- Optimal surgical visualization
- Reduced blood loss in a non-gravid uterus

Although data are limited, one review found that up to *26% of women did not conceive following TAC*, though the reasons were not investigated.

Early Pregnancy Cerclage (Late First to Early Second Trimester)

Advantages include:

- Exclusion of major fetal structural anomalies at the 11–13-week scan
- Opportunity for early aneuploidy screening

The ideal window for TAC placement is *14–15 weeks*, though SMFM suggests it may be safely performed up to *22 weeks' gestation*.

SURGICAL PROCEDURE (FIG. 1)

Preoperative Preparation

- Administer a single dose of a second-generation cephalosporin for prophylaxis.
- Insert a Foley catheter for continuous bladder drainage.

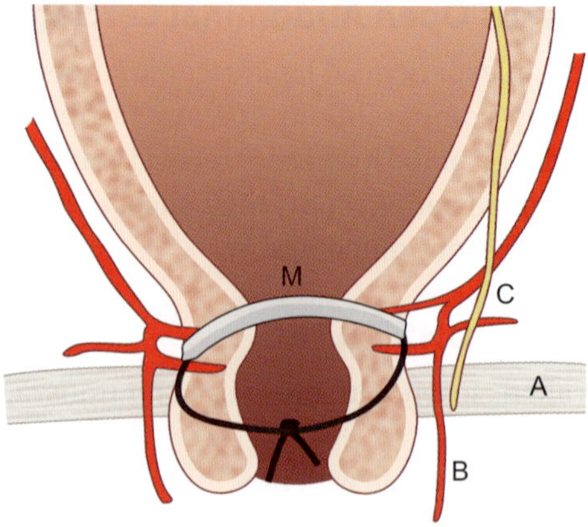

Fig. 1: Correct placement of the cervicoisthmic cerclage. (A: cardinal ligament; B: descending branch of uterine artery; C: a vascular space between ascending and descending branch of uterine artery; M: cerclage tape)

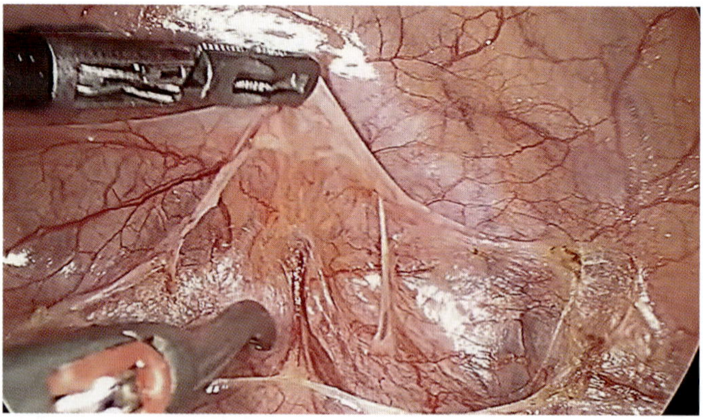

Fig. 2: Vesicouterine peritoneum being dissected to expose the cervicoisthmic junction.

Laparoscopic Technique

- General anesthesia is used, and the patient is placed in *dorsal lithotomy*.
- Pneumoperitoneum is typically created via *10 mm Visiport direct entry*, although in advanced gestations some prefer a Veress needle.
- Three 5-mm accessory ports are placed with adjustments according to gestational age.
- In interval cerclage, a vaginal manipulator may be used for optimal uterine mobilization. In a pregnant uterus, manipulation is done using atraumatic grasper or fan retractor.
- Dissection begins by opening the vesicouterine peritoneal fold to expose the lower uterine segment **(Fig. 2)**.
- The bladder is mobilized caudally, allowing visualization of the cervicoisthmic junction and uterine vessels **(Fig. 3)**.

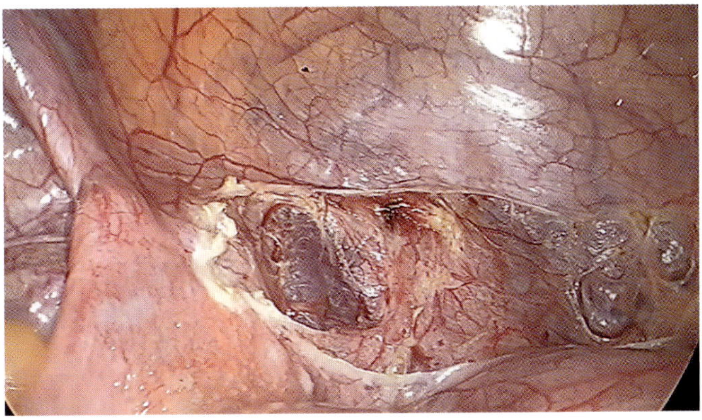

Fig. 3: Engorged uterine vessels at the level of internal os in a gravid uterus.

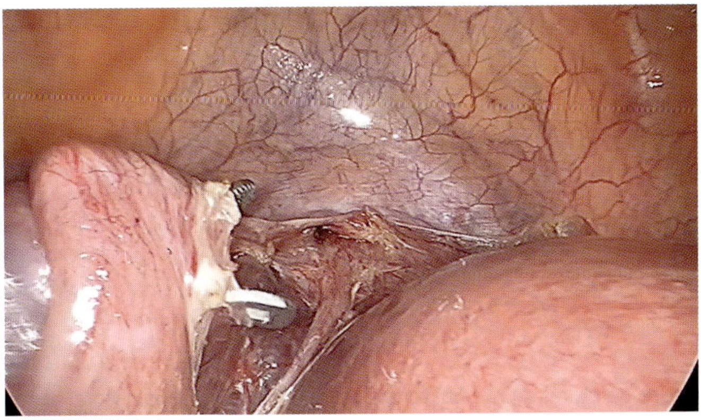

Fig. 4: Broad ligament window being created at the cervicoisthmic junction in the avascular space.

- In non-pregnant patients, manipulation of the uterus—including anteversion, retroversion, and slight rotation—may assist passage of the needle. In a pregnant uterus, bilateral broad ligament windows are opened to assist passage of needle with minimal manipulation of the uterus **(Figs. 4 and 5)**.
- A 5-mm Mersilene tape with a single needle is passed around the cervicoisthmic junction.
- Needle is passed at the level of internal os (uterovesical fold) from anterior to posterior on left side and posterior to anterior on right side, maintaining proximity to the uterosacral ligaments and ensuring placement medial to the uterine vessels but lateral to the cervix **(Figs. 6 to 9)**.
- Care must be taken to avoid excessively lateral insertion, which risks injury to the uterine vessels, or overly medial passage, which may pierce the cervix.

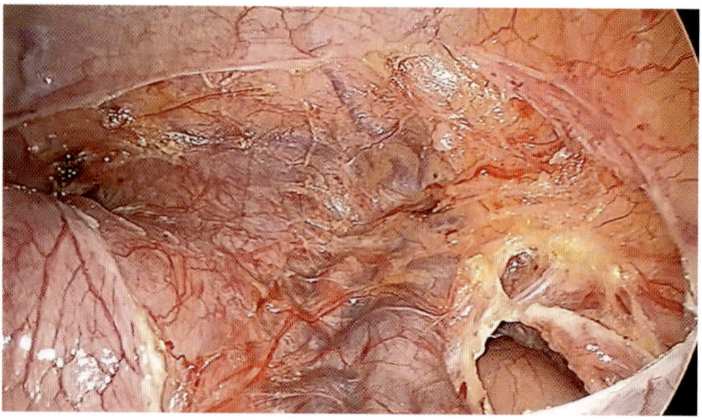

Fig. 5: Broad ligament window created bilaterally.

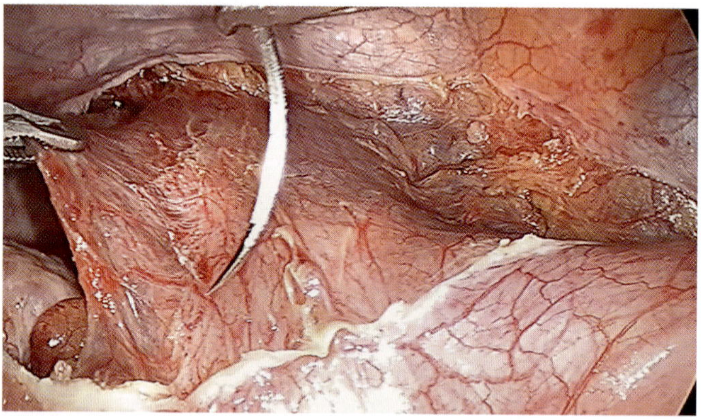

Fig. 6: Suture being taken medial to the blood vessels and just lateral to the cervix.

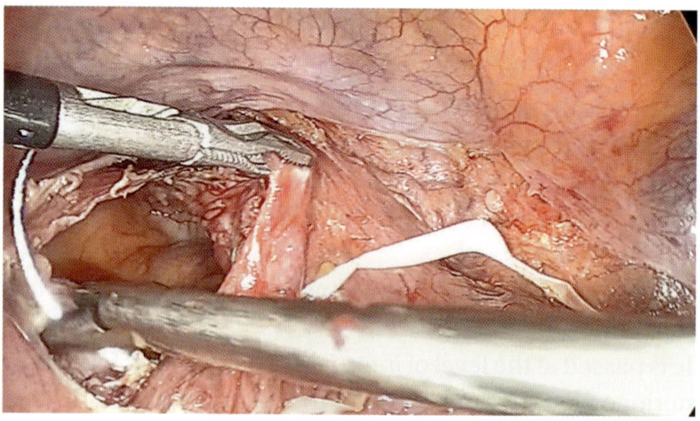

Fig. 7: Needle being drawn out from the broad ligament window ipsilaterally.

- The knot is tied anteriorly, although posterior tying is also acceptable. The knot is buried beneath the peritoneum to minimize bladder irritation **(Fig. 10 to 12)**.

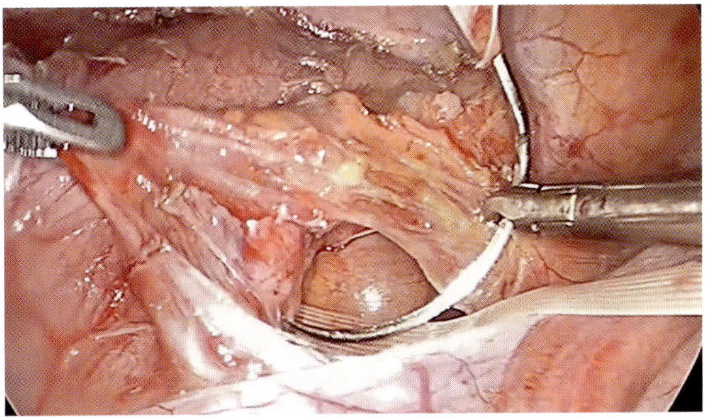

Fig. 8: Cerclage needle being brought from the contralateral broad ligament window posterior to anteriorly.

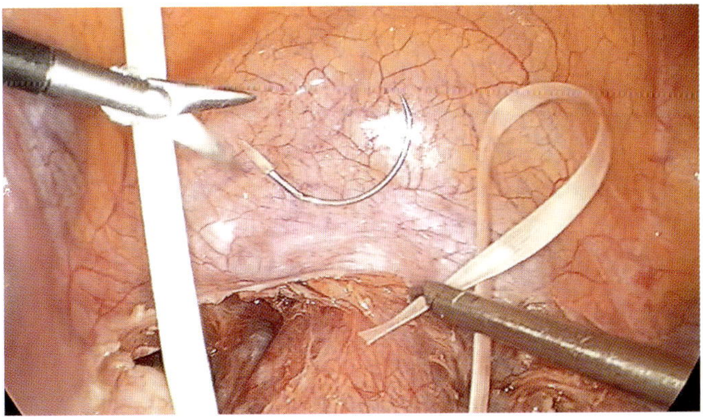

Fig. 9: Needle being cut and both ends of the tape brought anteriorly after ensuring the straightening of the tape at posterior end of uterus.

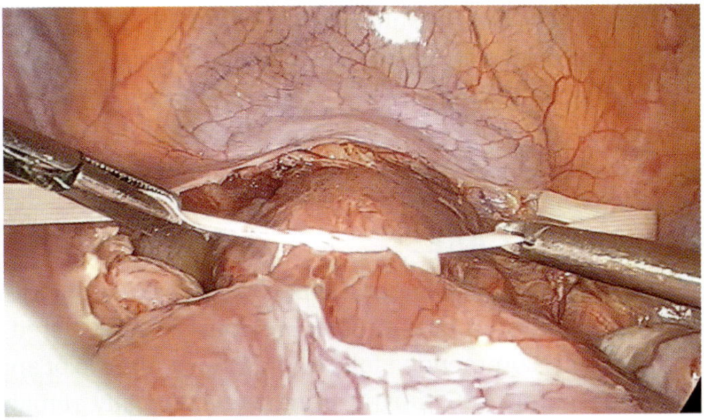

Fig. 10: Surgical knot being tied anteriorly at the cervicoisthmic junction with Mersilene tape.

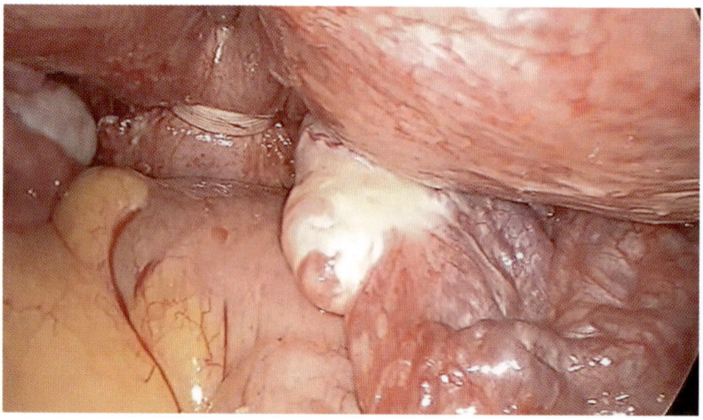

Fig. 11: Posterior view of the Mersilene tape at the level of uterosacral ligaments.

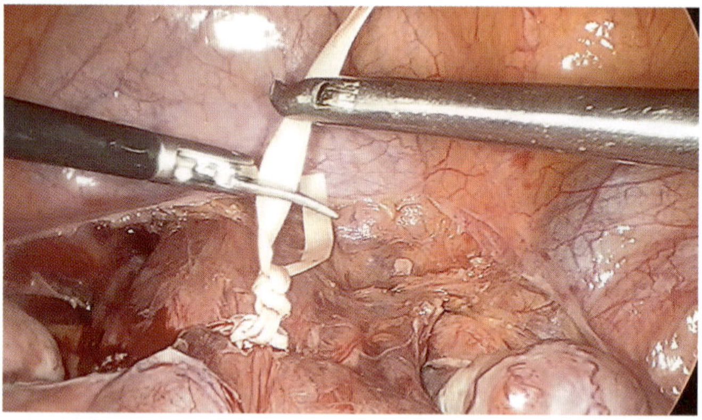

Fig. 12: Extra ends of the tape being cut after securely tying knots.

- The vesicouterine peritoneum is closed with a running *1-0 Vicryl or Monocryl* suture.
- Broad ligament windows are sutured with a *1-0 Vicryl* **(Fig. 13)**.
- Postoperative ultrasound confirms correct placement of the suture at the internal os **(Figs. 14A and B)**.

We will demonstrate surgical steps of laparoscopic abdominal cerclage in the following **Figures 2 to 14** with each step description following the image.

POSTOPERATIVE CARE

Routine postoperative management includes analgesia and antibiotics as required. Hydroxyprogesterone caproate, previously administered in some centers, is no longer recommended following FDA withdrawal of approval.

Patients undergoing TAC during pregnancy typically remain in the hospital for *approximately 2 days*. Assessment of *fetal cardiac activity* prior to discharge is common practice for reassurance.

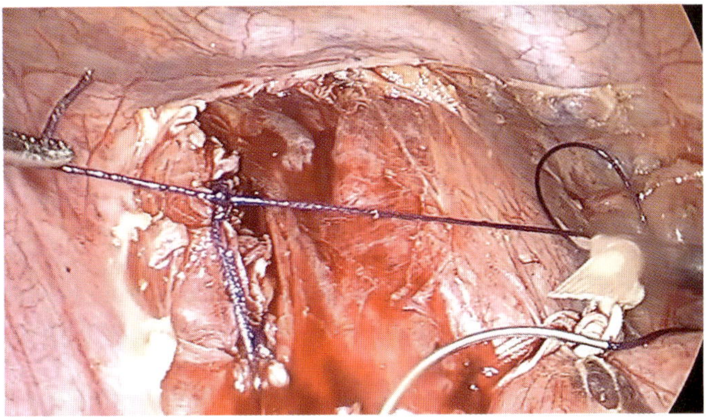

Fig. 13: Bilateral broad ligament windows being closed using absorbable Vicryl 1-0 suture.

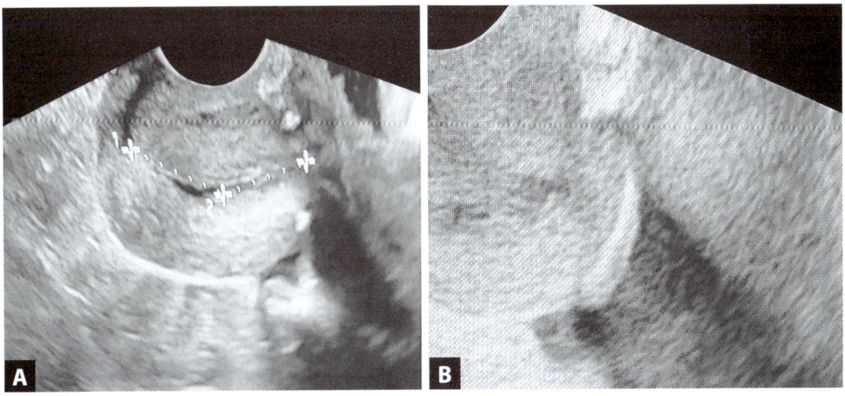

Figs. 14A and B: Postoperative ultrasound image demonstrating the placement of the cerclage at the level of internal os; (A) sagittal view, (B) transverse view.

Long-term follow-up follows standard obstetric surveillance. *Post-cerclage progesterone supplementation or serial cervical length monitoring is not recommended.*

SMFM advises *planned cesarean delivery between 37+0 and 39+0 weeks.* At cesarean, delivery is via a hysterotomy incision placed *above the cerclage,* which is left in situ for future pregnancies.

COMPLICATIONS

Potential complications include:

- Intraoperative blood loss
- Chorioamnionitis
- Wound infection
- Fetal loss within two weeks of surgery
- Preterm prelabor rupture of membranes

SUGGESTED READING

1. ACOG Practice Bulletin No.142: Cerclage for the management of cervical insufficiency. Obstet Gynecol. 2014 Feb;123(2 Pt 1):372-379.
2. Ades A, Parghi S, Aref-Adib M. Laparoscopic transabdominal cerclage: outcomes of 121 pregnancies. Aust N Z J Obstet Gynaecol. 2018;58:606-11.
3. Alfirevic Z, Stampalija T, Medley N. Cervical stitch (cerclage) for preventing preterm birth in singleton pregnancy. Cochrane Database Syst Rev. 2017; 6:CD008991.
4. Benson RC, Durfee RB. Transabdominal cervico uterine cerclage during pregnancy for the treatment of cervical incompetency. Obstet Gynecol. 1965;25:145-55.
5. Brown R, Gagnon R. Delisle MF. No. 373 cervical insufficiency and cervical cerclage. J Obstet Gynaecol Can. 2019;41(2):233-47.
6. Davis G, Berghella V, Talucci M, Wapner RJ. Patients with a prior failed transvaginal cerclage: a comparison of obstetric outcomes with either transabdominal or transvaginal cerclage. Am J Obstet Gynecol. 2000;183:836-9.
7. Drakeley AJ, Quenby S, Farquharson RG. Mid-trimester loss–appraisal of a screening protocol. Hum Reprod. 1998;13:1975-80.
8. Fick AL, Caughey AB, Parer JT. Transabdominal cerclage: can we predict who fails? J Matern Fetal Neonatal Med. 2007;20:63-7.
9. Han Y, Li M, Ma H, Yang H. Cervical insufficiency: a noteworthy disease with controver sies. J Perinat Med. 2020;48:648-55.
10. Lotgering FK, Gaugler-Senden IP, Lotgering SF, Wallenburg HC. Outcome after transabdominal cervicoisthmic cerclage. Obstet Gynecol. 2006;107:779-84.
11. McDonald IA. Cervical cerclage. Clin Obstet Gynaecol 1980;7:461-79.
12. Riiskjaer M, Petersen OB, Uldbjerg N, Hvidman L, Helmig RB, Forman A. Feasibility and clinical effects of laparoscopic abdominal cerclage: an observational study. Acta Obstet Gynecol Scand. 2012;91:1314-8.
13. Roman A, Suhag A, Berghella V. Cerclage: Indications and Patient counseling. Clin Obstet Gynecol. 2016;59:264-9.
14. Shennan A, Chandiramani M, Bennel P, et al. MAVRIC: a multicenter randomized controlled trial of transabdominal vs transvaginal cervical cerclage. Am J Obstet Gynecol. 2020;222:261.e1-9.
15. Shennan A, Story L, Jacobsson B, Grob man WA. FIGO good practice recommendations on cervical cerclage for prevention of preterm birth. Int J Gynaecol Obstet. 2021;155(1):19-22.
16. Society for Maternal-Fetal Medicine (SMFM); Temming L, Mikhail E; SMFM Publications Committee. Electronic address: pubs@smfm.org. Society for Maternal-Fetal Medicine Consult Series #65: Transabdominal cerclage. Am J Obstet Gynecol. 2023;228(6):B2-B10.
17. Sperling JD, Dahlke JD, Gonzalez JM. Cerclage use: a review of 3 national guidelines. Obstet Gynecol Surv. 2017;72:235-41.
18. Zaveri V, Aghajafari F, Amankwah K, Han nah M. Abdominal versus vaginal cerclage after a failed transvaginal cerclage: a systema\c review. Am J Obstet Gynecol. 2002;187:868-72.